Mental Health Information for Teens

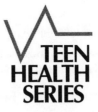

TEEN HEALTH SERIES

First Edition

Mental Health Information for Teens

Health Tips about Mental Health and Mental Illness

Including Facts about Anxiety, Depression, Suicide, Eating Disorders, Obsessive-Compulsive Disorders, Panic Attacks, Phobias, Schizophrenia, and More

◆

Edited by Karen Bellenir

Omnigraphics

615 Griswold Street • Detroit, MI 48226

Bibliographic Note

Because this page cannot legibly accommodate all the copyright notices, the Bibliographic Note portion of the Preface constitutes an extension of the copyright notice.

Edited by Karen Bellenir

Teen Health Series

Karen Bellenir, *Managing Editor*
David A. Cooke, MD, *Medical Consultant*
Joan Margeson, *Research Associate*
Dawn Matthews, *Verification Assistant*
Jenifer Swanson, *Research Associate*

Omnigraphics, Inc.

Matthew P. Barbour, *Vice President, Operations*
Laurie Lanzen Harris, *Vice President, Editorial Director*
Kevin Hayes, *Production Coordinator*
Thomas J. Murphy, *Vice President, Finance and Controller*
Peter E. Ruffner, *Senior Vice President*
Jane J. Steele, *Marketing Coordinator*

Frederick G. Ruffner, Jr., Publisher

Library of Congress Cataloging-in-Publication Data

Library of Congress Cataloging-in-Publication Data

Bellenir, Karen.
    Mental health information for teens / Karen Bellenir.
       p. cm. -- (Health reference series ; #)
    Includes bibliographical references and index.
    ISBN 0-7808-0442-2
    1. Teenagers--Mental health. 2. Adolescent psychology. 3. Child mental health. I. Title. II. Series.

RJ499 .B425 2001
616.89'00835--dc21

                                                   2001036364

∞

This book is printed on acid-free paper meeting the ANSI Z39.48 Standard. The infinity symbol that appears above indicates that the paper in this book meets that standard.

Printed in the United States

Table Of Contents

Preface ix

Part I: Mental Health Concerns

Chapter 1—You And Mental Health: What's The Deal? 3
Chapter 2—Self-Esteem 11
Chapter 3—Making Peace With Your Body 17
Chapter 4—Sadness: Is It Normal? 25
Chapter 5—Getting Along With Others 29
Chapter 6—Peer Pressure 31
Chapter 7—Controlling Anger... Before It Controls You 35
Chapter 8—A Teenager's Guide To Surviving Stress 45
Chapter 9—Is It Love? 51
Chapter 10—Love Doesn't Have To Hurt 55
Chapter 11—Physical And Emotional Abuse 69
Chapter 12—The Impact Of Divorce On Teenagers 73
Chapter 13—Teens And Grief 83
Chapter 14—When Your Parent Has A Mental Illness 89
Chapter 15—Information For Brothers And Sisters Of People
              With Mental Disorders 93

Part II: Common Types Of Mental Illness

Chapter 16—Mental, Emotional, And Behavior Disorders:
              An Overview 99
Chapter 17—Dealing With The Depths Of Depression 107

Chapter 18—Seasonal Affective Disorder 117

Chapter 19—Bipolar Disorder 121

Chapter 20—Early-Onset Bipolar Disorder 127

Chapter 21—Anxiety Disorders 147

Chapter 22—Generalized Anxiety Disorder 177

Chapter 23—Panic Disorder 181

Chapter 24—Phobias 193

Chapter 25—Social Phobia 203

Chapter 26—Post-Traumatic Stress Disorder 215

Chapter 27—Obsessive-Compulsive Disorder 219

Chapter 28—Computer Addiction 225

Chapter 29—Personality Disorders 229

Chapter 30—Attention Deficit Disorder 235

Chapter 31—Eating Disorders 241

Chapter 32—Body Dysmorphic Disorder 247

Chapter 33—Self-Injury 253

Chapter 34—Delusions And Delusional Disorders 267

Chapter 35—Schizophrenia 275

Part III: Suicide

Chapter 36—Teenage Suicide 285

Chapter 37—Depression And Substance Abuse
Can Be A Lethal Combination 293

Chapter 38—Thought Patterns That Predict Suicide Attempts 297

Chapter 39—Questions Teens Often Ask About
The Why And How Of Suicide 303

Chapter 40—Fifteen Myths About Teen Suicide 307

Chapter 41—If You Are Feeling Suicidal 317

Chapter 42—How To Prevent Suicide 321

Part IV: Getting Treatment

Chapter 43—Guidelines For Seeking Mental Health Care 327

Chapter 44—How Service Agencies Can Help You 335

Chapter 45—How To Find Help Through Psychotherapy 337

Chapter 46—How To Start A Self-Help/Advocacy Group 343
Chapter 47—Medications Used In Treatment 353
Chapter 48—What About St. John's Wort? 363

Part V: If You Need More Information

Chapter 49—Mental Health Resources 373
Chapter 50—Resources For Alcoholism And Substance Abuse 381

Index 391

Preface

About This Book

Depression—it's not just for adults. Some studies suggest that as many as one in eight teens suffer from major depression. Untreated, depression can lead to trouble in school, substance abuse, and even suicide. In fact, according to the National Institute on Mental Health, suicide is currently the leading cause of death among adolescents. And, teens aren't immune to other types of mental health disorders, including anxiety disorders (such as panic disorder, phobias, and post-traumatic stress syndrome), eating disorders, and psychotic illnesses. Some experts say that one in five young people are affected by mental health problems at any given time.

Tragically, an estimated two-thirds of all young people with mental health problems are not getting the help they need. Although people may be quick to notice signs of physical illness, the warning signs of mental illness often go unrecognized. This book provides teens with needed information about the causes of mental health problems, warning signs, and treatment options. It also provides tips on such topics as developing a positive self image, making and keeping friends, understanding emotional development, handling anger and stress, and overcoming trauma. Directories of resources, including toll-free telephone numbers and Internet addresses, are also provided.

How To Use This Book

This book is divided into parts and chapters. Parts focus on broad areas of interest. Chapters are devoted to single topics within a part.

Part I: Mental Health Concerns describes the components of mental health. It presents information about coping with normal life stresses and explains when unhealthy coping strategies may indicate mental illness. Other specific concerns, such as self-esteem, peer pressure, anger, love, abusive relationships, and grief are also addressed. Two chapters provide special information for teens who have family members with mental health disorders.

Part II: Common Types Of Mental Illness provides information about specific types of mental disorders, including depression, bipolar disorder, anxiety disorders, panic disorder, phobias, post-traumatic stress disorder, obsessive-compulsive disorder, personality disorders, attention deficit disorder, eating disorders, self-injury, delusional disorders, and schizophrenia. Individual chapters highlight the characteristics of the disorders, explain diagnostic procedures, and provide information about treatment issues.

Part III: Suicide focuses on the problem of suicide in adolescents. It includes statistical information along with facts about the links among depression, substance abuse, and suicide. Separate chapters offer answers to commonly asked questions about suicidal practices and dispel popular myths. Practical help for suicide prevention is also included.

Part IV: Getting Treatment provides information about seeking treatment for mental health disorders. It explains the differences among the various types of agencies and professionals who provide mental health care services, and it describes common fees and practices. Medications frequently used in conjunction with psychotherapy are also explained.

Part V: If You Need More Information provides a directory of mental health resources, including verified contact information and, where available, toll-free telephone numbers, hotlines, and Internet information. Because many adolescent mental health disorders are linked to substance abuse, a separate directory of resources for alcoholism and substance abuse is also provided.

Bibliographic Note

This volume contains documents and excerpts from publications issued by the following government agencies: Center for Mental Health Services (CMHS), National Center for Complementary and Alternative Medicine

(NCCAM), National Institute of Mental Health (NIMH), and the U.S. Food and Drug Administration (FDA).

In addition, this volume contains copyrighted documents and articles produced by the following organizations and journals: American Psychological Association, American School Health Association's *Journal of School Health*, Anxiety Disorders Association of America, *Brown University Child and Adolescent Behavior Letter*, Butler Hospital, Child and Adolescent Bipolar Foundation, Children's Hospital for Teens (Akron, Ohio), Clinical Reference Systems, Columbia University, Depression and Related Affective Disorders Association, Focus Adolescent Services, *Harvard Mental Health Letter*, Manisses Communications Group, National Alliance for the Mentally Ill (NAMI), National Mental Health Association, National Mental Health Consumer's Self-Help Clearinghouse, Nemours Foundation, Nidus Information Services, Inc., self-injury.net, Suicide Information and Education Centre (SIEC), Suite 101.com, Inc., TAG: Teen Age Grief, Inc., *The Addiction Letter*, University of Illinois at Urbana-Champaign/Counseling Center, and Weekly Reader Corporation's *Current Health 2*.

Full citation information is provided on the first page of each chapter. Every effort has been made to secure all necessary rights to reprint the copyrighted material. If any omissions have been made, please contact Omnigraphics to make corrections for future editions.

Acknowledgements

In addition to the organizations listed above, special thanks are due to researchers Jenifer Swanson and Joan Margeson, verification assistant Dawn Matthews, permission specialists Maria Franklin and Carol Munson, and editorial assistants Buffy Bellenir and Mike Bellenir.

Note From The Editor

This book is part of Omnigraphics' *Teen Health Series*. The series provides basic information about a broad range of medical concerns. It is not intended to serve as a tool for diagnosing illness, in prescribing treatments, or as a substitute for the physician/patient relationship. All persons concerned about medical symptoms or the possibility of disease are encouraged to seek professional care from an appropriate health care provider.

At the request of librarians serving today's young adults, the *Teen Health Series* was developed as a specially focused set of volumes within Omnigraphics' *Health Reference Series*. Each volume deals comprehensively with a topic selected according to the needs and interests of people in middle school and high school. If there is a topic you would like to see addressed in a future volume of the *Teen Health Series*, please write to:

Editor
Teen Health Series
Omnigraphics, Inc.
615 Griswold Street
Detroit, MI 48226

Our Advisory Board

The *Teen Health Series* is reviewed by an Advisory Board comprised of librarians from public, academic, and medical libraries. We would like to thank the following board members for providing guidance to the development of this series:

Dr. Lynda Baker, Associate Professor of Library and Information Science, Wayne State University,
Detroit, MI

Nancy Bulgarelli, William Beaumont Hospital Library,
Royal Oak, MI

Karen Imarasio, Bloomfield Township Public Library,
Bloomfield Township, MI

Karen Morgan, Mardigian Library, University of Michigan-Dearborn
Dearborn, MI

Rosemary Orlando, St. Clair Shores Public Library,
St. Clair Shores, MI

Medical Consultant

Medical consultation services are provided to the *Teen Health Series* editors by David A. Cooke, MD. Dr. Cooke is a graduate of Brandeis University, and he received his M.D. degree from the University of Michigan. He completed residency training at the University of Wisconsin Hospital and Clinics. He is board-certified in Internal Medicine. Dr. Cooke currently works as part of the University of Michigan Health System and practices in Brighton, MI. In his free time, he enjoys writing, science fiction, and spending time with his family.

Part 1

Mental Health Concerns

Chapter 1

You And Mental Health: What's The Deal?

Life can be tough, especially when you're a teenager. These years that are filled with challenges and adventures are also filled with many worries and problems: pressures to win, to be liked, to do well in school, to get along with your family, to get over break-ups, and to make important decisions about your life. Most of these stresses are unavoidable and worrying about them is natural. But pay attention if you're feeling extremely sad, hopeless, or worthless. Maybe you haven't felt this way, but a friend has. These and other warning signs could signal a mental health problem. This book will tell you more about mental health, how to know when there might be an overwhelming problem, what to do about it, and where to get help.

Question: I'm fine. My friends are fine. So why do I need to know about this?

Mental health problems can happen to people of any age, race, or religion or from any kind of family—no matter what kind of job, education, or income level. ANYONE. What you learn now may be useful later for yourself or someone you know. You can help reduce people's fears and lack of understanding by sharing what you've learned—that mental health problems are real and that people with mental health problems can and should get help.

About This Chapter: The main text in this chapter is taken from "You and Mental Health: What's the Deal?" a brochure produced by the U.S. Department of Health and Human Services, Substance Abuse and Mental Health Services Administration; DHHS Publication No. (SMA) 95-3073, February 1995.

Question: What is mental health?

Mental health is how you think, feel, and act in order to face life's situations. It is how you look at yourself, your life, and the people in your life; how you evaluate your options and make choices. Mental health includes things like handling stress, relating to other people, and making decisions. And like many physical aspects of your health, it develops as you get older.

Everyone has mental health. Mental health ranges from good to not so good and even to poor. A person's mental health may move through the range; sometimes a person is healthier than at other times and sometimes he or she needs help to handle problems. Many people experience mental health problems at some time during their lives.

Question: What are mental health problems?

Mental health problems are real. They affect your thoughts, body, feelings, and behavior. Doctors call some of them:

- depression

- bipolar or manic-depressive illness

- attention deficit hyperactivity disorder (ADHD)

- anxiety disorders

- eating disorders

- schizophrenia

- conduct disorder

✎ **Weird Words**

Mental Health: A state of mind in which a person is able to maintain satisfactory relationships with other people and to cope with the stresses of daily living.

These disorders are not just a passing phase; they can really interfere with a person's life. Mental health problems can be severe and can lead to school failure, loss of friends, or family problems.

Question: What causes these problems?

Mental health problems in young people are caused by biology, environment, or a mix of both. If young people are exposed to violence, loss of important people, abuse, or neglect, then they are more likely to be at risk for mental health problems. Other risk factors may include feeling continuous rejection because of race, religion, sexual orientation, or family income. Schools, families, and communities can probably prevent some mental health problems by protecting young people from these extremely stressful kinds of environmental factors. And when there are problems, seeking help early may prevent them from getting worse.

Mental health problems are not your fault. They don't mean you are weak or a failure. They don't mean you aren't trying. Whatever the cause, the important thing is to get help.

Question: What are some warning signs of a mental health problem?

There are many different signs that may point to a possible problem. Some of them are included in the list below. Pay attention if you (or your friends):

Are troubled by feeling:

- really sad and hopeless without good reason and the feelings don't go away.
- very angry most of the time, cry a lot, or overreact to things.
- worthless or guilty a lot.
- anxious or worried a lot more than other kids.
- unable to get over a loss or death of someone important.
- extremely fearful—you have unexplained fears or more fears than most kids.
- constantly concerned about physical problems or physical appearance.
- like your mind is being controlled or is out of control.

Experience big changes in the way you get along; for example you:

- do much worse in school.
- lose interest in things you usually enjoy.
- have unexplained changes in sleeping or eating.
- avoid friends or family and want to be alone all the time.
- daydream so much you can't get things done.
- feel as if you can't handle life or consider suicide.
- hear voices talking to you or about you that you cannot explain.

Find yourself limited by:

- poor concentration—you can't think straight or make up your mind.

- being unable to sit still or focus your attention.

- worrying about being harmed, hurting others, or about doing something "bad."

- feeling like you have to wash, clean things, or perform certain routines hundreds of times a day in order to avoid danger.

- thoughts that race through your head—almost so fast you can't follow them.

- persistent nightmares.

♣ It's A Fact!!

For some, mental health means minding stress levels and striking a healthy balance between work and home. For those with mental disorders, it may mean learning to manage and overcome their illness. But, no matter who you are, mental health is far more than an absence of a mental illness; mental health is something all of us want for ourselves.

Mental health is determined by:

- How you feel about yourself
- How you feel about others
- How you meet the demands of everyday life

One way of explaining mental health is to describe characteristics of a mentally healthy person. There are many different degrees of mental health and no one characteristic is indicative of good mental health; nor can the lack of any one characteristic signify a mental illness. In fact, nobody has all the traits of good mental health all the time.

From: "Mental Health and You: A Mental Health Checklist," © 1998, revised February 2000 National Mental Health Association. Reprinted with permission from the National Mental Health Association (1-800-969-NHMA).

Behave in ways that cause you problems, for example:

- use alcohol or other drugs.
- eat large amounts of food and then make yourself vomit, abuse laxatives, or take enemas to avoid weight gain.
- continue to diet and/or exercise obsessively although bone-thin.
- constantly violate the rights of others or break the law without regard for other people.
- do things that can be life-threatening.

Question: What helps?

Mental health problems are painful. They can hurt as much as (or more than) a serious physical injury. If you have a mental health problem, the sooner you get the right help, the sooner you may feel better. Some of the things that may help are:

- counseling
- family therapy
- group therapy
- crisis care
- behavior therapy
- special camp programs
- medications
- day treatment
- education programs
- tutoring

The people who help you should understand you and your family situation. They should talk about your strong points as well as your problems. And they should respect you and your feelings.

Question: How can I find help?

Find an adult you trust to talk to. This might be your parent, another relative, friend, neighbor, teacher, coach, member of the clergy, or family doctor. It's OK to ask for help. If one adult doesn't have answers, find someone who does.

You may also decide to get help from someone trained to support those with mental health problems, such as a:

- family doctor
- psychiatrist
- psychologist
- social worker
- special education teacher
- religious counselor
- school counselor
- nurse

✔ Quick Tip
A Mental Health Checklist

Do you feel good about yourself?

- I take pleasure in everyday things.
- I feel able to deal with most situations and am not overwhelmed by emotions.
- I can take life's disappointments in stride.
- I have a tolerant attitude toward myself as well as others.
- I am realistic about my abilities.
- I can accept my own shortcomings and laugh at myself.

Do you feel comfortable with other people?

- I am able to love and consider the interests of others.
- I have personal relationships that are satisfying and lasting.
- I can trust others and feel they can trust me.
- I do not take advantage of others nor do I let others take advantage of me.
- I feel a sense of responsibility to others.

Are you able to meet life's demands?

- I do something about problems as they arise.
- I accept responsibilities.
- I shape my environment when possible and adjust to life's challenges.
- I plan ahead and do not fear the future.
- I welcome new experiences and set realistic goals for myself.

From: "Mental Health and You: A Mental Health Checklist," © 1998, revised February 2000 National Mental Health Association. Reprinted with permission from the National Mental Health Association (1-800-969-NHMA).

Examples of where these people may work are:

- clinics or private offices

- schools

- social service agencies

- community mental health centers

- health maintenance organizations (HMOs)

Or you can call a local hotline. Call telephone directory assistance to get a local hotline number.

Question: What should I do if I think a friend has a mental health problem?

Encourage your friend to talk to a trusted adult. If he or she won't, you should talk with an adult you trust. If your friend talks about suicide, talk to an adult immediately. Don't go it alone. But above all, hang in there. Continue to be a friend. Listening to and being open to another person's feelings are important. Your friend doesn't need blame or shame. He or she needs your friendship.

Question: What if I want more information?

For free information about mental health—including publications, references, and referrals to local and national resources—call the National Mental Health Services Knowledge Exchange Network at 1-800-789-2627.

Chapter 2

Self-Esteem

What's The Meaning?

Self-esteem. So what does it mean? "Self" —that's easy. That's you! "Esteem" —this word is a bit trickier. It is not a word that most teenagers use on a daily basis. If you look it up in the dictionary, you will find: "Esteem— to hold in high regard" which means "to really like a lot. " For example, you really like your best friend, you really like your favorite teacher, or you really like your family. You get the picture. These are people you trust, respect, and enjoy spending time with.

So, let's look at the word "self-esteem" again: Self (you) -esteem (to like a lot) ... means you really like yourself a lot, both inside and out ... how you look as well as what you believe in.

Sometimes it's easy to like who you are. You feel great when you ace a test, score the winning goal, or tell a funny joke that everyone laughs at. But, how do you feel about yourself when you just said something mean or when you think you got a bad haircut? You start wishing you were someone else or that you could change how you look. You think you aren't good enough ... in school, on the team, or for the cool crowd. This is "low" or "negative" self-esteem.

About This Chapter: The text in this chapter is taken from "Teen Self-Esteem: Feeling Good About Yourself," © 1997, revised February 2000, National Mental Health Association. Reprinted with permission from the National Mental Health Association (1-800-969-NHMA).

Self-esteem ... means you like yourself ... all the time, not just when
things are going great! The good
news is you can learn to like yourself or have positive self-esteem all
the time. You are the one in control; you can make the difference.
But sometimes, you let others tell you
how to feel about yourself. From the day you
were born, your family, then your teachers and friends, have been influencing
your decisions. TV shows and music videos tell you what to wear and how to
act. Your music and magazines tell you how to feel and how to look.

> ❖ **It's A Fact!!**
>
> Positive self-esteem gives you the
> courage to be your own person.

What's The Importance?

So why is it important to have positive self-esteem if everyone is going to
tell you what to do, what to wear, and what to think? As a teenager, you now
have more responsibility to choose between right and wrong. You become
accountable for your actions. Positive self-esteem gives you the courage to be
your own person and to believe in your own values when the pressure is on to
make a big decision.

Your friends can put a lot of pressure on you. You want to be part of a
group or crowd. The crowd may be the "cool" crowd, the "jock" crowd, or the
"brainy" crowd. Belonging to a crowd is a part of growing up, learning to be
a friend, and learning about the world around you. It's OK to want to be
liked by others. But not when it means giving into pressure. Your friends are
now making many of their own decisions. And their decisions may or may
not be good for you.

It's never worth doing things that could hurt you or someone else. For
instance, drinking alcohol or using other drugs, having sex before you are
ready, joining a gang, or quitting school can all lead to trouble.

Think about what can happen if you give in to the wrong decision. Drinking or doing drugs and driving can lead to serious injury or death. Sex may
lead to pregnancy, STDs (sexually transmitted diseases) or AIDS. Joining a

gang may lead to illegal behavior and maybe jail. And quitting school takes away your best chance to be successful later in life.

It is not always going to be easy to stick to your values, but you will be happier if you do.

Only you know what is best for you. If you let your friends think for you, you won't be working toward your personal goals for your future. When you value and respect yourself, it keeps you from making bad decisions that may affect the rest of your life.

♣ **It's A Fact!!**

Do You Know These Answers?

1. Is it easy to change your self-esteem?

No. It means taking some time to understand who you are—what you like, don't like, feel comfortable with, and what goals you have. Ask for help from your parents, a school counselor, and your friends to find the answers. This takes time and hard work. It's a life-long process, but it's worth the work!

2. Does self-esteem guarantee success?

Success in school? Success playing sports or a musical instrument? Success with friends? No, but if you keep trying and doing your best, you are a success. Remember, having positive self-esteem will help you to achieve what you want. But when you don't succeed, it helps you to accept the situation and move on.

3. Does positive self-esteem mean "being stuck-up, snobby or on an ego trip"?

No. Kids who act this way usually are trying to pretend they are something they are not. In fact, they often have low self-esteem.

4. Can I help others feel good about themselves?

Yes. Don't put others down for how they feel, look or act. Be patient with your friends and family when they fall short. We all make mistakes from time to time.

✔ Quick Tip

How To Find Yourself

The teenage years can be a challenge because it is the time when young people discover what's important to them, how they should act, and how they fit into their group of friends. Sometimes you may "try out" different groups to see where you fit the best. You may choose a group of friends because that group is identified as being "tough" or "smart" or "athletic." Eventually you will find a group that you like, one that thinks like you, and does things that you like to do. This is better than trying to fake your way through friendships, because eventually people will find out what you are really like, and leave you alone.

You probably work very hard to keep everyone in your life happy with you: parents, friends, and a boyfriend or girlfriend. Sometimes this is not an easy thing to do. You may not be able to do all the things people expect of you. It is much better for you to follow what you know to be right and to do those things that will help you to achieve the goals you set for your life.

You may have heard people talking about "finding myself" or "getting to know who I am." What they are talking about is feeling comfortable with the way they act and the way they get along with other people. This has a lot to do with finding your "style" of doing things, and this usually happens while you are a teenager. Some people are quiet most of the time and others seem to talk a lot; some people like to do things fast, others like to take their time. There is almost an endless list of ways that people are different.

You may want to be like someone important in your life such as your parents or friends, and you may try to act like they do. You may also have some idea how kids who are the same race, religion, or class as you should act, and you will try to act the same. There is nothing wrong with patterning your life after someone else's, as long as you feel comfortable with it and you don't get into trouble just because it seems like the thing to do.

The choice of friends is an important part of adolescence. Of all the people you will come in contact with, perhaps none are more influential than your friends. The choices that you make are, therefore, very important. Choose a group that will lead you in the direction that you want to go. Do not expect that you alone will be able to fight any negative influences you see in your friends.

You are now faced with some very important decisions. You want to be independent from Mom and Dad, while at the same time you need their help and support. You also want to get along with them because through it all you still care for them and they still love you. It's best to let them know what you are thinking, and try to find some middle ground.

You may (or perhaps you already have) become more interested in sex—an adult issue that carries with it a lot of responsibility. What you decide to do and how you decide to act may not only affect what you think of yourself, it may also change your life in ways that you didn't expect.

How do you decide what choices to make? Some of it is through trial and error, discovering where your strengths lie and what your weaknesses are. Here are some tips to help you choose:

- Begin to focus on your strengths and things that you really are interested in.

- Set expectations that are realistic for you and that are based not only on what makes you happiest immediately but also what will make you happy in the long run.

- If there are actions or behaviors that make you feel guilty, sad, or angry, then that is a sign that these things are not in your best interest. It is best to pursue those things that will make you feel happy with yourself and satisfied that you've accomplished something.

- Take care of yourself physically. Your body is growing and your mind is growing as well. Things that you will do to yourself in the form of diets, exercise, drugs, alcohol and smoking all could have very long-lasting effects.

The thing to remember is that most adolescents get through these challenges, and chances are, you will too. Try to take care of yourself and make the decisions that you know are the right ones.

Source: "Self-Esteem," produced by Children's Hospital for Teens, Akron, Ohio; reprinted with permission.

How Do You Get Good Self Esteem?

OK. You think that having "positive" self-esteem is a good idea. How do you get it?

- Be honest with yourself. Figure out what your strengths and weaknesses are. Don't beat yourself up over your weaknesses. Don't compare yourself to others. Learn to accept yourself.

- Set realistic goals for yourself. Try to get the most out of your strengths without demanding or expecting too much of yourself. Take one day at a time. Do your best each day.

- Trust your own feelings. Listen to yourself. Pay attention to your emotions.

- Enjoy yourself when you have achievements. Celebrate your successful efforts. Don't downplay them.

☞ Remember!!

Feeling good about yourself helps you to:

- *Accept challenges.* Try a new sport or audition for the school play. And if you don't make the varsity team or get the lead in the play, you will at least enjoy trying and learning more about yourself.

- *Enjoy your life.* Happy people are fun to be around. A happy outlook helps you to make and keep new friends.

- *Believe in yourself.* If you think you can do something, you are more likely to do it.

- *Stay flexible.* Life is changing all the time. You can't stop it, but you can learn to live with it.

Chapter 3

Making Peace With Your Body

In this world of super-hunks and airbrushed beauties, finding fault with normal bodies has become a national pastime. Here's how to hold your head high and think the best of yourself—whatever your body's shape.

Many teens suffer from what the experts call "negative body image"—they don't like their bodies. And they're letting their thoughts about their bodies shatter their self-esteem, their sense of how valuable they are as people.

"I find it impossible to ever be satisfied with my body," says Sarah, a high school senior from San Diego, California. "After each pound slips away, I still feel the need to be thinner."

Her friend Stephanie understands Sarah's dilemma. "All I see are models in magazines who look so perfect, and that's how I want to be," she says.

Sarah and Stephanie are not alone. Nearly two of every five teens who replied to a nationwide survey that appeared in *USA Weekend* [in 1997] said they would feel better about themselves if they lost weight or (among boys) bulked up. The survey, published in May 1998, discovered that nearly seven out of 10 respondents said they felt either "somewhat satisfied" or "not at all satisfied" with their looks.

About This Chapter: The text in this chapter is from "How to Make Peace with Your Body," by Cindy Maynard in *Current Health 2*, September 1998, Vol. 25, No. 1, p. 6(6), © 1998 Weekly Reader Corporation; reprinted with permission.

Tony, 14, probably would agree. "I feel sad because everyone calls me fat," he says. "I exercise and do push-ups to help me lose weight. The kids call me 'Fat Boy,' 'Fatso,' and stuff—and it makes me mad."

Sarah, Stephanie, and Tony take part in a weekly body image group held for adolescents at Mesa Vista Hospital in San Diego. They asked [to be identified] by first name only. The group began when teens expressed a need to discuss their feelings and perceptions about their bodies in a supportive forum.

In this media-driven age, it seems most people are dissatisfied with their bodies. Recent studies show that kids as early as third grade are concerned about their weight. But, with body shapes rapidly changing, teens are the most vulnerable. During teen years, there is a lot of pressure to fit in.

Mirror, Mirror

Girls, in general, tend to be overly concerned about weight and body shape, say psychologists. Many strive for the "perfect" body and judge themselves by their looks, clothes, and ability to stay cover-girl thin.

But boys don't escape either. Today's culture celebrates tough,

✎ Weird Words

Anorexia Nervosa: An eating disorder characterized by an aversion to eating, excessive fasting, extreme and sometimes life-threatening weight loss, and fear of being fat. Anorexia nervosa is most often diagnosed in adolescent girls, and it is frequently accompanied by a distorted body image, feelings of being fat even if the patient is very thin, excessive activity, and amenorrhea (absence of menstruation).

Binge Eating Disorder: An eating disorder characterized by secretive episodes of uncontrolled eating in which large amounts of food are eaten in a short time. Unlike builima nervosa, the eating episodes are not followed by self-induced vomiting or other means of purging.

Bulimia Nervosa: An eating disorder characterized by repeated, secretive episodes of binge eating followed by self-induced vomiting, laxative abuse, or excessive exercise to avoid gaining weight. Periods of bulimic behavior can alternate with periods of normal eating or fasting.

muscular, and well-sculpted males. So naturally, boys are concerned with the size and strength of their body. They think they have to be "real" men. Yet many admit being confused as to what's expected of them. This confusion can make it harder than ever to feel good about themselves. It's not surprising that sports such as wrestling, boxing, and gymnastics (which demand top conditioning) contribute to a negative body image. The need to make weight for a sport often leads to eating problems.

But boys like Jon Maxwell, 15, say sports make them feel better about themselves. "Guys are in competition, especially in the weight room," Jon says. "One will say, 'I can bench 215 pounds,' and the other guy says, 'Well, I can bench 230 pounds.' If you're stronger, you're better."

Daniel Schaufler, age 16, agrees. "Guys are into having the perfect body," he says. "If you feel good about your body, you automatically feel good about yourself."

Mission Impossible

Most of our cues about what we should look like come from the media, parents, and peers. This constant obsession with weight, the size of our body, and longing for a different shape or size can be painful.

Most teens watch an average of 22 hours of TV a week and are deluged with images of fat-free bodies in the pages of health, fashion, and teen magazines, according to Eva Pomice in her book, *When Kids Hate Their Bodies*. The result: Many try to achieve this "look," which is an impossible goal. As a result, many teens intensely dislike their bodies.

Take a look at the most popular magazines on the newsstands. Psychologist David M. Garner says in a recent *Psychology Today* article: "The media show an image of the perfect woman that is unattainable for somewhere between 98 and 99 percent of the female population." Remember: It's a career for these women; they're pros. Many have had major body makeovers and have full-time personal trainers. Photos in ads can be airbrushed or changed by computer. Body and facial imperfections, such as pimples, can be erased or changed at will.

The images of men and women in ads today have the power to make us feel bad about and lose touch with ourselves. Ads aren't intended to promote self-esteem or positive self-image. They're intended to sell products—and they do. In the United States, consumers spend billions of dollars to pursue the perfect body. The message "thin is in" is blasted at us thousands of times a day through TV, movies, magazines, billboards, newspapers, and songs. In a 1997 Body Image Survey, published by *Psychology Today*, teenagers reported that viewing very thin or muscular models made them feel insecure about themselves.

✔ Quick Tip

How do you feel about your body? When you look in the mirror, are you proud of what you see, or do you think, "I'm too short," "I'm too fat," or "If only I were thinner or more muscular"? Answer the following questions to determine how you view yourself.

1. Have you avoided sports or working out because you didn't want to be seen in gym clothes?

2. Does eating even a small amount of food make you feel fat?

3. Do you worry or obsess about your body not being small, thin, or good enough?

4. Are you concerned your body is not muscular or strong enough?

5. Do you avoid wearing certain clothes because they make you feel fat?

6. Have you ever disliked your body?

7. Do you feel bad about yourself because you don't like your body?

8. Do you want to change something about your body?

9. Do you compare yourself to others and "come up short"?

If you answered "Yes" to three or more questions, you may have a negative body image.

Parents can give mixed messages, too—especially if they're constantly dieting or have body or food issues of their own. How young people perceive and internalize these childhood messages about their bodies determines their ability to be confident about their appearance.

Slimming Down, Bulking Up

America's preoccupation with dieting has made the diet business a multibillion-dollar industry. And it put questionable diet drugs, such as fen-phen, on the market. Fenfluramine (Pondimin and Redux) diet pills were taken off the market [in 1997] because of their link to heart damage.

Just as bad, some student athletes who want to build strength are using danger-ous anabolic steroids or other hor-mones. These chemicals have serious side effects, and they can stunt growth and cause liver damage, cancer, and high blood pressure.

This intense focus on food, fat, and body building also can lead to abnormal eating habits—such as yo-yo dieting and compulsive eating—that can turn into eating disorders.

♣ It's A Fact!!

According to a nation-wide survey conducted by *USA Weekend,* nearly two of every five teens who replied said they would feel better about themselves if they lost weight or bulked up.

Eating disorders, such as anorexia and bulimia, aren't new. More than 100 years ago, the first case of anorexia nervosa, or self-induced starvation, was documented. The incidence of eating disorders, including compulsive overeating and dieting, continues to increase. The American Psychiatric As-sociation (APA) estimates that at any given time 500,000 Americans are battling eating disorders.

These disorders hit males and females in every area of society. More people became aware of them in 1995 when Princess Di began talking openly about her struggles with bulimia. Christy Henrich, a high-ranked gymnast, paid the high-est price. At the time of her death, she was 22 years old and weighed barely 50 pounds. Actress Tracey Gold still struggles with her eating disorder.

Body Image, Body Love

Psychologists and counselors recognize that a negative body image has a powerful impact on self-esteem, our assessment of our value as individuals. When we think about body image, generally we think about aspects of our physical appearance. But body image is much more. It is our mental picture of our bodies as well as of our thoughts, feelings, judgments, sensations, awareness, and behavior. It's part of our mental picture of our total selves—the picture that shapes the way we think about our value as people.

Feel bad about your body and in time you're likely to feel bad about other aspects of yourself. It's not uncommon for people who think poorly of their bodies to have problems in other areas of their lives—including relationships and careers. That's why it's so important, experts say, to avoid letting your body affect your self-esteem. Positive self-esteem, says the National Mental Health Association (NMHA), "means you really like yourself a lot, both inside and out...how you look as well as what you believe in."

Iris, age 18, who is currently at Montecatini, a residential treatment center for anorexia in La Costa, California, is working to raise her self-esteem. "I must work hard to keep my chin up, establish eye contact, and have the courage, honesty, and trust to say what I am feeling," she says. "I have a right to be heard and to give my opinion. That is one way I will accomplish self-respect and gain the same respect from others."

But you don't have to have an eating disorder to find achieving a healthy self-image a challenge. Here are some tips from the NMHA and elsewhere on how teens who are unhappy with their bodies can start feeling better about themselves.

Accepting Your Body

How can you learn to feel good and accept yourself no matter what your size or shape?

First step: When you look in the mirror, make sure you find at least one good point for every demerit you give yourself. Become aware of your positives.

Here are some other steps you can take to build a better body image—
and more positive self-esteem:

- Accept the fact that your body's changing. In the teen years, your body
  is a work in progress. Don't let every new inch or curve throw you off
  the deep end.

- Decide which of the cultural pressures—glamour, fitness, thinness,
  media, peer group—prevent you from feeling good about yourself. Then
  do something to counteract this. How about not buying magazines
  that promote unrealistic body images?

- Exercise. When you want to feel good about the way you look, exercise. It helps improve your appearance, health, and mood.

- Emphasize your assets. You have many. Give yourself credit for positive qualities. If there are some things you want to change, remember:
  Self-discovery is a lifelong process.

- Make friends with the person you see in the mirror. Say "I like what I
  see. I like me." Do it until you believe it.

- Question ads. Instead of saying "What's wrong with me?" say "What's
  wrong with this ad?" Write the company. Set your own standards instead of letting the media set them for you.

- Ditch dieting and the scale. These are two great ways to develop a
  healthy relationship with your body and weight.

- Challenge size bigotry and fight size discrimination whenever you can.
  Don't speak of yourself or others with phrases like "fat slob" or "thun-
  der thighs."

- Be an example to others by taking people seriously for what they say,
  feel, and do rather than how they look.

- Accepting yourself is the starting point. Monique, age 18, in treatment for an eating disorder in La Costa, California, says she has learned
  to feel better about her body and herself. She has become more appre-
  ciative of those "inner qualities that make up who I am, such as my
  creativity, my intuition, and my self-motivation." At the same time,

she has learned to block out "the negative thoughts based on my distorted body image, such as being too fat, never good enough for anyone, including myself."

☞ Remember!!

You can't exchange your body for a new one. The best you can do is find peace with the one you have. Your body is where you're going to be living for the rest of your life. Isn't it about time you made it your home?

Chapter 4

Sadness: Is It Normal?

Feeling down? Got the blues? You're not alone. Everyone gets sad (yes, everyone you ever met). Sad feelings can happen pretty often, too—over half of teenagers go through a sad period at least once a month.

When you're sad, it feels like it will last forever, but usually feelings of sadness don't last very long—a few hours, or maybe a day or two. It's important to recognize when sadness does not go away, because this may mean there is a more serious problem, called depression.

What Is Sadness?

When you're sad, the world seems dark and unfriendly. You have a hurt deep inside that crushes your heart and your spirit. Many times you cry, and the tears are hard to stop. Crying usually makes you feel better. When sadness starts to go away, it feels like a heavy blanket is being lifted from your heart.

When Is It Natural To Feel Sad?

Feeling sad every once in a while is natural. Maybe you didn't get something you really wanted. Maybe you miss somebody. Maybe somebody you really like rejected you, and you don't feel so great about yourself. There are lots of reasons that people feel sadness. These are some of them:

Loss is the most common cause of sadness. It's a very sad thing to lose someone or something that you care about. There are many kinds of loss. The death of a relative, friend, or pet can bring weeks or months of sad feelings. Other kinds of loss can also bring sadness, like people close to you getting a divorce or moving to a new town and leaving old friends. With this sadness, you might also feel angry or guilty, like you may have caused the loss—but you probably did not. Sometimes it is hard to think straight because you cannot get your mind off your loss. Usually, the load of sadness you carry after a loss will lighten over time, although there may always be a little bit of sadness left.

♣ It's A Fact!!

Here are some of the signs and symptoms that can be seen with depression:

- feeling anxious, "empty," or "numb"
- feeling hopeless, like there's nothing to look forward to
- feeling guilty or worthless
- feeling lonely or unloved
- loss of interest in regular activities—things are not fun anymore
- difficulty concentrating in school and when doing homework—sometimes school grades fall
- difficulty concentrating on other activities, like reading or watching TV—not remembering what a book or a TV show was about
- having less energy and feeling tired all the time
- sleeping too much or not enough
- not eating enough (smaller appetite) and weight loss, or eating too much (bigger appetite) and weight gain
- thoughts about death—sometimes attempts at suicide
- spending less time with friends and more time alone
- frequent crying, often for no obvious reason
- feeling irritable (every little thing gets on your nerves)
- feeling restless (being unable to sit still or relax)
- physical complaints, such as dry mouth, dry skin, difficulty having bowel movements, headaches, stomach or chest pain, vomiting, dizziness

Relationships bring happiness and fun most of the time, but they can also bring sad times. Many kids fight with family members, especially their parents, in the struggle to grow up and gain independence. They fight about things like money, clothing, haircuts, school, friends, and cars. In school, problems with teachers and grades may cause periods of sadness as well. Other kids, both friends and enemies, can cause hurt feelings and sadness through fighting, teasing, peer pressure, not giving you support, or leaving you out of group activities.

Self-image, the way you feel about yourself, can be a big reason for sad feelings. Most people, even adults, are not completely happy with the way they look. Many people feel that they are not as good as they would like to be in sports or in school. And lots of people feel shy when talking to other people (especially with members of the opposite sex).

When Is Sadness A Problem?

If sad feelings go on for too long, it's called depression.

People who have depression may not know it. Often it's a parent or teacher who notices behavior changes. Sometimes depression can occur for no obvious reason. Sometimes it runs in families. Other times there is an apparent reason, like a long period of sadness after the loss of someone really close, such as a parent; problems at home, including, violence, illness, divorce, or alcohol or drug use; child abuse or neglect; rape; and long-term illness, burns, or accidents.

It is very important for people who have depression to get help. When they do, they can get better very quickly. Sometimes treatment involves talking to someone who knows all about depression. Sometimes it means taking medications. Sometimes both of these things are used.

If you think you have depression, or you just have sadness that simply will not go away, it is important to talk to an adult about it: a parent, relative, doctor, teacher, guidance counselor, coach, minister, or close adult friend. This person can help find the right type of treatment. Many cities also have mental health hot lines or suicide hotlines that are listed in the phone book. There is always somebody to talk to—somebody who can help.

☞ **Remember!!**

If you have persistent sadness or if you think you have depression, there are people who want to help you. If you don't know who to talk to, the following organizations can help you find some-one:

National Hospital for Kids in Crisis
5300 KidsPeace Dr.
Orefield, PA 18069
Toll-Free: 800-446-9543
Fax: 610-799-8801
Website: http://www.kidspeace.org

National Institute of Mental Health
6001 Executive Boulevard, Rm. 8184, MSC 9663
Rockville, MD 20892-9663
Toll-free 800-64-PANIC (647-2642)
Website: http://www.nimh.nih.gov

The National Mental Health Association
1021 Prince St.
Alexandria, VA 22314-2971
Toll-Free: 800-969-6642
Website: http://www.nmha.org

Chapter 5

Getting Along With Others

Relationships with the people in our lives are very important to all of us. How we get along with parents, brothers and sisters, friends, and boyfriends or girlfriends, helps determine how well we feel about ourselves and the world. While each of these relationships is unique, some things about all of them are the same.

For starters, all relationships require good communication. Being able to communicate with others is probably the most important skill for developing and keeping good relationships. A good way to learn good communication is to practice a communication technique call "active listening."

The first step in active listening is making sure you look directly at the person while he or she is talking. That is called eye contact. Eye contact lets the person know that you are really paying attention.

The second step is learning to use "I" statements instead of "you" statements. For example, when you feel angry with someone say, "I feel angry when you do that," instead of "You make me angry." "You" statements make people feel like they are being accused and make it harder to communicate.

About This Chapter: The text in this chapter is from "Getting Along With Others," produced by Children's Hospital for Teens, Akron, Ohio; reprinted with permission.

The third step in active listening is making sure you have understood what the person has said. You can do this by repeating in your own words what you think he has said. For example, tell the person, "It sounds to me like you are saying... ." Or ask the person, "Do you mean...?"

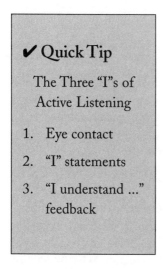

✔ Quick Tip

The Three "I"s of
Active Listening

1. Eye contact

2. "I" statements

3. "I understand ..."
    feedback

Another part of good communication is letting your feelings be known to others. It is not always easy to do. It means letting someone know what you want or what you expect. Sometimes expectations are quite clear. For instance, a teacher or coach expects you to accomplish certain work. You expect their guidance, leadership, and praise when the job is done well. Other times, expectations may be unclear. For example, you might really want to go to the movies with your boyfriend or girlfriend. If they don't call, you might feel angry and disappointed. The actual problem is that they just didn't know how much you wanted to go to the movies.

And finally, remember also that all relationships, even the good ones, have rocky times. Those times pass. Keep working on your good communication skills.

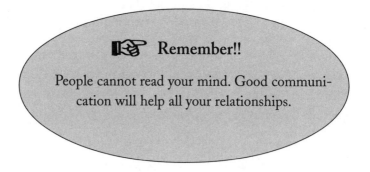

☞ Remember!!

People cannot read your mind. Good communication will help all your relationships.

Chapter 6

Peer Pressure

Peers are your friends, your equals, or someone in your age group you would like to be like. The importance of your peers to you is a natural part of adolescence. It is part of the growing process that occurs as your separate from your parents and begin to form your own identity. We as human beings seek approval. In the past you looked to your parents for approval. Now you look to your peers.

There are two kinds of pressures you deal with everyday:

- Pressures that come from **outside** of you, such as a dad who expects you to get an A in Physics because he wants you to be an engineer, or the heaviness you feel when your team's winning score depends on you.

- Pressures that come from **inside** of you, such as being pushed around by a peer whom you have accepted. You can only be forced to approve standards which you have chosen to approve. You are the only one who makes the decision about who will be your peers and how much you will follow them.

About This Chapter: The text in this chapter is from " Peer Pressure," produced by Children's Hospital for Teens, Akron, Ohio; reprinted with permission.

The only real way to deal with peer pressure is to first deal with yourself. If you have confidence in your own judgments, specific life goals, and are convinced about what is right and wrong for you, you will not feel pressured as much by peers. It is when you are not sure of where you stand that you feel the pressure of the group. To grow up means to develop the ability to set your own standards of proper conduct, right or wrong, and your life goals. Be prepared to be pushed around by the shifting standard of others if you have not taken the time and energy to make your own judgments. It is an ongoing struggle to achieve this, but it is well worth it.

✔ Quick Tip

The following strategies can help you avoid negative peer pressure:

- Identify a helpful role model
- Have personal goals
- Good communication with friends
- Take responsibility for your decisions and your life

How can you take a step toward overcoming the forces shoving at your life? It does take time and energy to form your identity so that you can avoid being a victim of peer pressure. The following steps can help:

- **Choose someone you would like to be like**—don't just look at your immediate peers. Other kids are in the same stage as you, and you won't be a teenager all your life. Choose someone farther along such as a coach, teacher, youth leader at your church or synagogue, even an older sister or brother, or parent. Talk to the person you admire. Ask them how they made choices. Ask them for helpful advice. Be careful that instead of a "popular figure," your person is a person who admits mistakes as well as successes.

- **Set your goals.** Do you know where you are going? Do you know how you will get there? Some of us know from a very young age what we want to do with our lives. Others just drift along until they are finally nudged into a direction by outside forces. Don't be afraid to make some definite decisions about your future; later in life you can always change them. Use your admired person as a counselor when setting your goals. He/she can help give you the direction into goals that are possible for you. You don't want to let this person make decisions for you. Instead let them help you learn how to make good decisions and choices. People who want to overcome peer pressure and be an individual have decided where they are going.

- **Talk about your pressured feelings with your friends.** You are not the only one feeling these pressures and fears. Talking to friends about your feelings can help alleviate loneliness and depression.

- **Make a decision to take full responsibility for your life**—all of us, even grown-ups, wish someone else could be responsible for us like it was when we were young children. But the hardest part of being an adult is to assume that your life is your own and you must take control of what becomes of it. You are growing into an adult each day. You can make decisions that show that you are in charge.

As you learn to be responsible for yourself, you'll find that you will develop skills to be more involved with others. If you don't want things forced on you, you'll develop an inner strength that is your own, not based on the ideas about you from someone else. You will work to develop your own life goals, direction, values and standards.

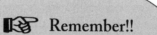 Remember!!

Peer pressure has been around a long time. Everyone of every age has to learn to deal with it. Either you will have control of it or it will have control of you. But you can have the challenge and reward of shaping your own life.

Chapter 7

Controlling Anger ... Before It Controls You

We all know what anger is, and we've all felt it: whether as a fleeting annoyance or as a full-fledged rage.

Anger is a completely normal, usually healthy, human emotion. But when it gets out of control and turns destructive, it can lead to problems: problems at school or at work, in your personal relationships, and in the overall quality of your life. And it can make you feel as though you're at the mercy of an unpredictable and powerful emotion. This chapter is meant to help you to understand and get a handle on handling anger.

What Is Anger?

The Nature Of Anger

Anger is "an emotional state that varies in intensity from mild irritation to intense fury and rage," according to Charles Spielberger, Ph.D., a psychologist who specializes in the study of anger. Like other emotions, it is accompanied by physiological and biological changes; when you get angry, your heart rate and blood pressure go up, as does the level of your energy hormones, adrenaline and noradrenaline.

Anger can be caused by both external and internal events. You could be angry at a specific person (such as a teacher, coworker, or supervisor) or event (a grade, a traffic jam, a canceled flight), or your anger could be caused by worrying or brooding about your personal problems. Memories of traumatic or enraging events can also trigger angry feelings.

Expressing Anger

The instinctive, natural way to express anger is to respond aggressively. Anger is a natural, adaptive response to threats; it inspires powerful, often aggressive, feelings and behaviors, which allow us to fight and to defend ourselves when we are attacked. A certain amount of anger, therefore, is necessary to our survival.

On the other hand, we can't physically lash out at every person or object that irritates or annoys us; laws, social norms and common sense place limits on how far our anger can take us.

People use a variety of both conscious and unconscious processes to deal with their angry feelings. The three main approaches are expressing, suppressing, and calming.

Expressing your angry feelings in an assertive—not aggressive—manner is the healthiest

✎ Weird Words

Hypertension: Abnormal high blood pressure (usually defined as more than 140/90).

Imagery: A therapeutic technique in which the patient learns to use the imagination to substitute pleasant thoughts for unpleasant ones associated with anxiety or to divert attention from pain.

Pathological: Pertaining to a disease, a disease process, or caused by a disease, especially related to changes in body tissue structure or function.

Physiological: Relating to the functions and activities of living organisms.

Relaxation: Reducing tension.

Yoga: A system of exercises and physical postures aimed at promoting control of the body, mind, and breath.

way to express anger. To do this, you have to learn how to make clear what your needs are, and how to get them met, without hurting others. Being assertive doesn't mean being pushy or demanding; it means being respectful of yourself and others.

Anger can be suppressed, and then converted or redirected. This happens when you hold in your anger, stop thinking about it and focus on something positive. The aim is to inhibit or suppress your anger and convert it into more constructive behavior. The danger in this type of response is that if it isn't allowed outward expression, your anger can turn inward—on yourself. Anger turned inward may cause hypertension (high blood pressure) or depression.

Unexpressed anger can create other problems. It can lead to pathological expressions of anger, such as passive-aggressive behavior (getting back at people indirectly, without telling them why, rather than confronting them head-on) or a personality that seems perpetually cynical and hostile. People who are constantly putting others down, criticizing everything and making cynical comments haven't learned how to constructively express their anger. Not surprisingly, they aren't likely to have many successful relationships.

Finally, you can calm yourself down inside. This means not just controlling your outward behavior but also controlling your internal responses, taking steps to lower your heart rate, calm yourself down and let the feelings subside.

As Dr. Spielberger notes, "when none of these three techniques work, that's when someone—or something—is going to get hurt."

Anger Management

The goal of anger management is to reduce both your emotional feelings and the physiological arousal that anger causes. You can't get rid of, or avoid, the things or the people that enrage you, nor can you change them, but you can learn to control your reactions.

Are You Too Angry?

There are psychological tests that measure the intensity of angry feelings, how prone to anger you are and how well you handle it. But chances are good that if you do have a problem with anger, you already know it. If you find yourself acting in ways that seem out of control and frightening, you might need help finding better ways to deal with this emotion.

Why Are Some People More Angry Than Others?

According to Jerry Deffenbacher, Ph.D., a psychologist who specializes in anger management, some people are really more "hotheaded" than others; they get angry more easily and more intensely than the average person. There are also those who don't show their anger in loud spectacular ways but are chronically irritable and grumpy. Easily angered people don't always curse an throw things; sometimes they withdraw socially, sulk, or get physically ill.

People who are easily angered generally have what some psychologists call a low tolerance for frustration, meaning simply that they feel that they should not have to be subjected to frustration, inconvenience, or annoyance. They can't take things in stride, and they're particularly infuriated if the situation seems somehow unjust: for example, being corrected for a minor mistake.

♣ **It's A Fact!!**
Some people show their anger by behaving in a "hotheaded" manner; some are chronically irritable and grumpy. Other people don't show their anger directly, but instead withdraw socially, sulk, or even get physically sick.

What makes these people this way? A number of things. One cause may be genetic or physiological; there is evidence that some children are born irritable, touchy, and easily angered, and that these signs are present from a very early age. Another may be sociocultural. Anger is often regarded as negative; we've taught that it's all right to express anxiety, depression, or other emotions but not to express anger. As a result, we don't learn how to handle it or channel it constructively.

Research has also found that family background plays a role. Typically, people who are easily angered come from families that are disruptive, chaotic, and not skilled at emotional communications.

Is It Good To "Let It All Hang Out"?

Psychologists now say that this is a dangerous myth. Some people use this theory as a license to hurt others. Research has found that "letting it rip" with anger actually escalates anger and aggression and does nothing to help you (or the person you're angry with) resolve the situation.

It's best to find out what it is that triggers your anger, and then to develop strategies to keep those triggers from topping you over the edge.

What Strategies Can You Use To Keep Anger At Bay?

Relaxation

Simple relaxation tools such as deep breathing and relaxing imagery can help calm down angry feelings. There are books and courses that can teach you relaxation techniques, and once you learn them you can call upon them in any situation. If you are involved in a relationship where both partners are hot-tempered, it might be a good idea for both of you to learn these techniques.

Some simple steps you can try:

- Breathe deeply, from your diaphragm; breathing from your chest won't relax you. Picture your breath coming up from your "gut."

- Slowly repeat a calm word or phrase such as "relax," "take it easy." Repeat it to yourself while breathing deeply.

- Use imagery; visualize a relaxing experience, from either your memory or your imagination.

- Non-strenuous, slow yoga-like exercises can relax your muscles and make you feel much calmer.

Practice these techniques daily. Learn to use them automatically when you're in a tense situation.

Cognitive Restructuring

Simply put, this means changing the way you think. Angry people tend to curse, swear, or speak in highly colorful terms that reflect their inner thoughts. When you're angry, your thinking can get very exaggerated and overly dramatic. Try replacing these thoughts with more rational ones. For instance, instead of telling yourself, "oh, it's awful, it's terrible, everything's ruined," tell yourself, "it's frustrating, and it's understandable that I'm upset about it, but it's not the end of the world and getting angry is not going to fix it anyhow."

Be careful of words like "never" or "always" when talking about yourself or someone else. "This machine never works," or "You're always forgetting things" are not just inaccurate. They also serve to make you feel that your anger is justified and that there's no way to solve the problem. They also alienate and humiliate people who might otherwise be willing to work with you on a solution.

For example, you have a friend who is constantly late when you make plans to meet. Don't go on the attack; think instead about the goal you want to accomplish (that is, getting you and your friend there at about the same time). So avoid saying things like, "You're always late! You're the most irresponsible, inconsiderate person I have ever met!" The only goal that accomplishes is hurting and angering your friend.

State what the problem is, and try to find a solution that works for both of you; or take matters into your own hands by, for instance, setting your meeting time a half-hour earlier so that your friend will, in fact, get there on time, even if you have to trick him or her into doing it! Either way, the problem is solved and the friendship isn't damaged.

Remind yourself that getting angry is not going to fix anything, that it won't make you feel better (and may actually make you feel worse).

Logic defeats anger, because anger, even when it's justified, can quickly become irrational. So use cold hard logic on yourself. Remind yourself that the world is "not out to get you," you're just experiencing some of the rough spots of daily life. Do this each time you feel anger getting the best of you, and it'll help you get a more balanced perspective.

Angry people tend to demand things: fairness, appreciation, agreement, willingness to do things their way. Everyone wants these things, and we are all hurt and disappointed when we don't get them, but angry people demand them, and when their demands aren't met their disappointment becomes anger. As part of their cognitive restructuring, angry people need to become aware of their demanding nature and translate their expectations into desires. In other words, saying "I would like" something is healthier than saying "I demand" or "I must have" something. When you're unable to get what you want, you will experience the normal reactions—frustration, disappointment, hurt—but not anger. Some angry people use this anger as a way to avoid feeling hurt, but that doesn't mean the hurt goes away.

Problem-Solving

Sometimes, our anger and frustration are caused by very real and inescapable problems in our lives. Not all anger is misplaced, and often it's a healthy, natural response to these difficulties. There is also a cultural belief that every problem has a solution, and it adds to our frustration to find out that this isn't always the case. The best attitude to bring such a situation, then, is not to focus on finding the solution but rather on how you handle and face the problem.

Make a plan, and check your progress along the way. (People who have trouble with planning might find a good guide to organizing or time management helpful.) Resolve to give it your best, but also not to punish yourself if an answer doesn't come right away. If you can approach it with your best intentions and efforts, and make a serious attempt to face it head-on, you will be less likely to lose patience and fall into all-or-nothing thinking, even if the problem does not get solved right away.

Better Communication

Angry people tend to jump to—and act on—conclusions, and some of those conclusions can be pretty wild. The first thing to do, if you are in a heated discussion, is to slow down and think through your responses. Don't say the first thing that comes into your head, but slow down and think carefully about what you want to say. At the same time, listen carefully to what the other person is saying and take your time before answering.

Listen, too, to what is underlying the anger. For instance, you like a certain amount of freedom and personal space, and your "significant other" wants more connection and closeness. If he or she starts complaining about your activities, don't retaliate by painting you partner as a jailer, a warden, or an albatross around your neck.

It's natural to get defensive when you're criticized, but don't fight back. Instead, listen to what's underlying the words: the message may be that this person might feel neglected and unloved. It may take a lot of patient questioning on your part, and it may require some breathing space, but don't let your anger—or a partner's—let a discussion spin out of control. Keeping your cool can keep the situation from becoming a disastrous one.

Using Humor

"Silly humor" can help defuse rage in a number of ways. For one thing, it can help you get a more balanced perspective. When you get angry and call someone a name or refer to them in some imaginative phrase, stop and picture what that word would literally look like. If you're at work and you think of a co-worker as a "dirt-bag" or a "single-cell life form," for example, picture a large bag full of dirt (or an amoeba) sitting at your colleague's desk, talking

---

✔ **Quick Tip**

Some Other Tips For Easing Up On Yourself

- *Timing*: If you and your parents tend to fight when you discuss things at night—perhaps you're tired, or distracted, or maybe it's just habit—try changing the times when you talk about important matters so these talks don't turn into arguments.

- *Avoidance*: If it isn't important, don't make yourself look at what infuriates you. The point is to keep yourself calm.

- *Finding alternatives*: If your one of your daily routines leaves you in a state of rage and frustration, give yourself a project—find another alternative way of accomplishing your goals.

on the phone, going to meetings. Do this whenever a name comes into your head about another person. If you can, draw a picture of what the actual thing might look like. This will take a lot of the edge off your fury; and humor can always be relied on to help un-knot a tense situation.

The underlying message of highly angry people, Dr. Deffenbacher says, is "things oughta go my way!" Angry people tend to feel that they are morally correct, that any blocking or changing of their plans is an unbearable indignity, and that they should NOT have to suffer this way. Maybe other people do, but not them.

When you feel that urge, he suggests, picture yourself as a god or goddess, a supreme ruler who owns the streets and stores and office space, striding alone and having your way in all situations while others defer to you. The more detail you can get into your imaginary scenes, the more chances you have to realize that maybe you are being a little unreasonable; you'll also realize how unimportant the things you're angry about really are.

There are two cautions in using humor. First, don't try to just "laugh off" your problems; rather, use humor to help yourself face them more constructively. Second, don't give in to harsh, sarcastic humor; that's just another form of unhealthy anger expression.

What these techniques have in common is a refusal to take yourself too seriously. Anger is a serious emotion, but it's often accompanied by ideas that, if examined, can make you laugh.

Changing Your Environment

Sometimes it's our immediate surroundings that give us cause for irritation and fury. Problems and responsibilities can weigh on you and make you feel angry at the trap you seem to have fallen into, and all the people and things that form that trap.

Give yourself a break. Make sure you have some "personal time" scheduled for times of the day that you know are particularly stressful. One example is the working mother who has a standing rule that when she comes home from work, the first fifteen minutes is brief quiet time. Then she feels better prepared to handle demands from her kids without blowing up at them.

Do You Need Counseling?

If you feel that your anger is really out of control, if it is having an impact on your relationships and on important parts of your life, you might consider counseling to learn how to handle it better. A psychologist or other licensed mental health professional can work with you in developing a range of techniques for changing your thinking and you behaviors.

When you talk to a prospective therapist, tell her or him that you have problems with anger that you want to work on, and ask about his or her approach to anger management. Make sure this isn't only a course of action designed to "put you in touch with your feelings and express them" —that may be precisely what your problem is.

With counseling, psychologists say, a highly angry person can move closer to a middle range of anger in about 8 to 10 weeks, depending on circumstances and the techniques used.

☞ **Remember!!**

You can't eliminate anger—and it wouldn't be a good idea if you could. In spite of all your efforts, things will always happen that will cause you anger. Life will always be filled with frustration, pain, loss, and the unpredictable actions of others. You can't change that; but you can change the way you let such events affect you. Controlling your angry responses can keep them from making you even more unhappy in the long run.

What About Assertiveness Training?

It's true that angry people need to learn to become assertive (rather than aggressive), but most books and courses on developing assertiveness are aimed at people who don't feel enough anger. These people are more passive and acquiescent than the average person; they tend to let others walk all over them. That isn't something most angry people do. Still, these books can contain some useful tactics to use in frustrating situations.

Chapter 8

A Teenager's Guide To Surviving Stress

Sometimes being a teenager is tough. Your parents expect a lot from you; you just flunked a biology test; your best friend is changing schools; and today, you are supposed to give a report in front of the class. Your heart is beating faster than usual. Your palms feel sweaty. Your stomach feels a little upset. What's going on? Guess what. You may be stressed out.

Stress—Good Or Bad?

Your mother is stressed about a big project at work. But she's excited. Your father is stressed taking care of your sick grandmother and working. He's tired and cranky. Can stress he good and bad? Yes.

Everyone feels stress during their lives, sometimes everyday. Stress (the excited feeling or cranky attitude) is your body's reaction to something you may or may not want to do. Feeling stress is normal. Sometimes stress is good. It keeps you focused and doing the best you can. Like the excitement before a game or getting ready for a dance. But sometimes stress feels bad. You can't sleep or feel sad and lonely. Don't ignore these feelings. Stress needs your attention. Take care of yourself. Get help.

About This Chapter: The text in this chapter is taken from "Teen Stress: A Teen's Guide to Surviving Stress," © 1997, revised February 2000, National Mental Health Association. Reprinted with permission from the National Mental Health Association (1-800-969-NMHA).

Signs Of Stress

Normally you are pretty cool about things. But some days you don't feel like your old self. Your mother is asking what's wrong and your best friend tells you "to get over it." But you just want them to leave you alone. Are you stressed out? Your body or your emotions will let you know.

So Why Are You Stressed Out?

It's different for everyone, but there are some common stressful situations like those listed below. Read the list. Can you relate to any of them?

- *Family problems*—these may include divorce, money problems, violence in the home, problems with alcohol or other drugs, or the illness or death of a family member or close friend.

♣ **It's A Fact!!**

Are you stressed out? Do you....

- Feel tired for no good reason?
- Have headaches or unexplained back pain?
- Eat a lot more or a lot less than you usually do?
- Have trouble sleeping?
- Have more colds than usual?
- Suddenly have flashes of anger or fight more with your family members and friends?
- Let little things bother you?
- Feel sad, moody, and lonely?
- Have trouble thinking as clearly as you usually do?

If you answered "yes" to any of these questions, you may be stressed out.

- *Peer pressure*—are your friends asking you to do things you don't want to do such as use alcohol or drugs, have sex, join clubs, or go places you don't want to go?

- *Self-esteem*—the way you feel about yourself emotionally or physically—do you think you aren't smart enough or as popular as you should be?

- *Your grades*—do you feel one test score will change your life?

- *Too many activities in your life*—trying to do a lot of things may sound like fun, but may not give you enough time to "chill out."

- *Changes in your everyday routine*—such as switching schools, moving to a new neighborhood, moving on to a new grade.

- *Fear of violence*—feeling unsafe in your neighborhood or school can create almost constant stress.

How Can You Beat Stress?

Chill out and take a break. Think about what's going on in your life. Remember you're in control. You may not be able to change the outside world, but you can learn to deal. Here are some tips for beating stress. (Share them with your parents. Maybe they can use some help too!)

- *Recognize that you are in charge of your stress.* You have control over a lot of your activities. You can choose to make changes in your life which reduce your stress.

- *Try to determine the importance of a situation.* Example: if you are not invited to a certain party it is not the end of the world. It may seem that way to you but, it's not. There *will* be other parties.

- *Go easy on yourself.* No one is perfect. No one gets it right all the time. No one always has all the answers. If you are trying hard and doing your best, that's all any one can ask of you. Give yourself credit.

- *Take one thing at a time and prepare for it!* Manage your time wisely. For example: if you have two big tests on Thursday, don't wait until Wednesday night to study for both of them. A little planning can go a long way to reducing stress.

- *Take care of yourself.* Eat healthy foods. Limit your intake of caffeine and get enough rest. Drugs and alcohol won't solve anything and may lead to bigger problems.

- *Exercise regularly.* Pick a physical activity you really like, not what you think others expect you to do.

✔ Quick Tip

Your Plan For Action

When your own stress signals tell you that you're feeling too much stress, try putting this four-step problem-solving plan into action:

1. Determine what's really causing the stress you feel.

2. "Brainstorm" for solutions. Think of as many you can, no matter how silly they seem. A trusted family member, teacher, or school counselor may have good ideas.

3. Talk about what may happen, the good things and the bad things, with all of your possible solutions.

4. Act. Make the best decision you can and follow through on your decision. If it still doesn't work for you, next time, try another solution. Don't be afraid to fail. Everyone makes mistakes. You may be embarrassed or disappointed that your solution didn't go exactly as you expected. This may not be comforting, but this happens to everyone at sometime. Next time, you will succeed!

- *Laugh or cry a little.* It may help to relieve your feelings and improve your outlook. It's not hard to do, and it can reduce stress. Remember, this too shall pass!

- *Get involved.* Join activities at school, at your church, or other activity center. For example, volunteer at a local animal shelter. You will feel better about yourself and build new friendships.

- *Relax.* Relaxing is essential for everybody's physical and mental health, and enriches your quality of life. Find out what really makes you relax and spend at least half an hour each day doing it. It might be curling up with a good book, going on a hike ride, or listening to your favorite music.

- *Visualize yourself doing the activity or being in the situation which is giving you stress.* Use your mind to "see" how you can manage a potentially stressful situation in advance. Whether it's a dreaded presentation or a challenging sports event, you may find that visual rehearsals boost self-confidence and lead to increased success, especially when you see yourself being great!

- *Don't suffer in silence.* An honest talk with someone you trust can help you get rid of bottled-up feelings and help you see things in a different light. Don't hesitate to go to your school counselor or a trusted adult for help. Knowing when to ask for help is a strength, not a weakness.

If you still need help, where do you go? It's important to remember that, whatever your problems, there are people and resources available to help. Try talking to a close friend, a trusted family member, teacher, or school counselor when you're upset. Not only will you find it a relief to talk about your problem, but you might learn there are caring people who want to help and support you.

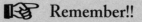 **Remember!!**

If you are feeling stressed out everyday for several weeks, you may have a more serious problem or situation on your hands. Speak to your parents or another adult immediately. Asking for help is not a sign of weakness. You are never too young or too old to ask for help.

Chapter 9

Is It Love?

What Is Love?

When you are a teenager, you find yourself experiencing a variety of new emotions. One of the most intense feelings during this period in your life may be romantic love.

Because of the newness of these emotions, many teenagers question whether the feelings they have now will last a lifetime. It is hard to be objective when feelings that you have never had before are so strong. It is almost impossible to imagine that you might not always care about the person that you love now. With all of these things in mind, it is easy to understand why teenagers have so many doubts and fears about whether the feeling they have will last.

Unfortunately, it is hard to place an age limit on love since it is a question of your maturity, not of your age. Some teenagers will share a love that lasts a lifetime, while others will share an intense emotional experience that lasts for a short time. Relationships often change as your self-image and emotional maturity change.

About This Chapter: The text in this chapter is from "Is This Love?" produced by Children's Hospital for Teens, Akron, Ohio; reprinted with permission.

Lack of experience and lack of complete maturity make many teenagers unable to give and share in a way that will build a lasting relationship. A mature, lasting love requires these elements:

- Confidence in yourself and your loved one

- Security whether you're alone or together

- Acceptance of each other's faults

- Attraction that's more than physical

- Ability to survive on your own

- Ability to handle responsibility

✎ **Weird Words**

Emotion: A strong feeling such as joy, anger, or fear, accompanied by psychological changes and arising without conscious effort; often demonstrated with alterations in behavior.

However, if you're clinging and possessive, idealizing the qualities of your loved one, caught up in the excitement and feelings of romance, dependent on physical attraction, and wrapped up in the life of your loved one, your relationship will probably end eventually. Infatuation cannot withstand pressure or time.

If your relationship does end, it may be hard to accept, but you'll be better off as a result. Breaking up is not the end of the world. Don't do anything crazy to hurt yourself or others. Talking out your hurts with a friend, parent, or adult who you trust can help.

In any case, realize that responsibility comes with love. You must be mature enough to accept obligations to yourself, your loved one, and your family. Sex adds even more responsibility to a relationship. An unplanned pregnancy and bad grades may not seem terrible right now, but could ruin the rest of your life. Sex alone cannot make a relationship work. Sex is not love. Sex is only an expression of love—and may not always be that.

Teenage marriages have an extremely high divorce rate. It is unrealistic to think that marriage may solve any problems that you have with your parents, in a relationship, or in school. For teens, marriage can create more problems than it solves with the expenses of rent, utilities, food, medical bills, insurance, taxes, and clothing. It holds enormous obligations.

Mature love is a commitment—wanting the best for that person. It is not selfish. It is fulfilling the needs of another and finding enjoyment through giving, not just taking. What does your relationship have going for it besides the physical aspect? If the physical aspect of your relationship were taken away would there be enough there to keep it going? There are different types of love. Physical desire is only one "feeling" of love. Love involves friendship and affection. The deepest love is that which is self-sacrificing. Some say "I love you if ..." or "I love you because..." Love at its deepest level says, "I love you in spite of ..."

Are You In Love?

Clearly, it is often difficult to decide whether you are really in love. When you are experiencing such intense emotions for the first time, it is hard to be objective. It seems that lasting relationships come with emotional maturity, not with age, and that permanent relationships should be entered into wisely and carefully. The most important thing is that you handle serious relationships with the responsibility they require.

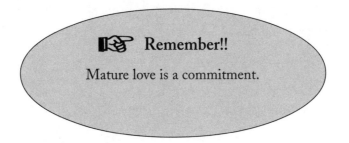

Remember!!

Mature love is a commitment.

Chapter 10

Love Doesn't Have To Hurt

Do These Scenes Sound Familiar?

Kevin is walking in the school hallway with his friends and sees his girlfriend at her locker with her friends. When he goes up to her, she gives him a cold look and says loudly, "I don't know why I even bother with you, loser! I guess I just keep you around because I feel sorry, for you." Kevin feels frustrated because he doesn't know what he did and embarrassed because his friends saw his girlfriend putting him down.

That kind of humiliation hurts, and it is a big deal.

Jennie and Tyrone lunch in the cafeteria with their friends. They start teasing each other, but then the playing turns to insults. Tyrone sees that Jennie is upset but doesn't stop. When Jennie gets up and says, "Get away from me, I hate you." Tyrone says, "Shut up" and slaps her across the face.

That slap is violence, and it is a big deal.

About This Chapter: Text in this chapter is from "Love Doesn't Have to Hurt Teens," © 1997 by the American Psychological Association. Reprinted with permission. The American Psychological Association developed this document with consultation from the Partners in Program Planning in Adolescent Health (PIPPAH), whose members include: American Bar Association's Center on Children and the Law and Commission on Domestic Violence, American Dietetic Association, American Medical Association, and the National Association of Social Workers.

Tony and Emily have been going out for a few weeks, and he is beginning to act like he owns her. He complains when she spends time with her best friend—or anyone except him. He expects her to meet him in the halls between classes, eat lunch with him, let him go home with her after school, and be with him every weekend. Afraid she'll lose him, Emily begins to cut herself off from her friends.

That kind of possessiveness isn't love—it is abuse, and it is a big deal.

Christine and Allison are in an intense argument. Christine gets madder and madder, until she finally grabs Allison, shakes her, and shoves her against the wall. Later, Christine apologizes, saying, "I'm not proud I lost my temper, but you really pushed my buttons. You should know better than to get up in my face like that, because you know I get too angry to control myself."

That kind of behavior—the shoving and then blaming someone else for the behavior—is violence, and it is a big deal.

Alfredo and Maria, who have been going out for a few weeks, are making out. Maria has been clear that she doesn't want to go any further than kissing, but Alfredo becomes aggressive, disregarding her request to slow down and back off. He forces her to have intercourse, later telling her she was a tease and was asking for it.

That kind of sex is rape and it is a big deal.

Love Shouldn't Hurt Like This

It's wonderful to be in love. It's exciting, romantic, and fun, and you feel like nothing can go wrong. Sure, like the love songs say, love hurts sometimes. You worry, and you wonder if the person you love really loves you, or if he or she is cheating on you. But knowing that *love hurts* doesn't mean you should expect to *get hurt*—to be put down, slapped, embarrassed in front of your friends, pushed, yelled at, forced to have sex if you don't want it, controlled by, or afraid of the person you're going out with.

Getting hurt like that isn't love. It's dangerous. It's violence. It can happen to anybody, even if you're smart or popular or strong or sophisticated.

And it doesn't matter who you're seeing. It happens to girls and to boys. It happens in same-sex relationships.

At first, if it happens to you or to a friend, you might not get what's going on. You're thinking, "I can handle this. I can make it stop"; or "There's no black eye. I'm not getting pushed down a stairway." "I shouldn't take put-downs so seriously." Maybe you're thinking, "He only gets jealous because he loves me." "She only slapped me to show attitude." "She won't love me if I don't do everything she wants, when she wants it." "To show my love, I should want to spend every spare moment with him."

Or maybe you do get it. You know things aren't right, but you feel alone. You're ashamed to tell your friends. You're afraid the explosions and jealousy will get worse if you tell anyone. You're afraid to tell your parents because

♣ It's A Fact!!

- Nearly one in 10 high school students will experience physical violence from someone they're going with. Even more teens will experience verbal or emotional abuse during the relationship.

- Between 10 and 25 percent of girls between the ages of 15 and 24 will be the victims of rape or attempted rape. In more than half of those cases, the attacker is someone the girl goes out with.

- Girls are not the only ones who are abused physically or emotion- ally in relationships. Boys also experience abuse, especially psy- chological abuse. Boys rarely are hurt physically in relationships, but when it happens, it's often severe. Boys also can be pressured or forced into unwanted sex, by girls or by other boys.

- Violence happens in same-sex relationships, too. When it does, gay and lesbian teenagers often don't know where to turn for help. If they are not comfortable telling people that they're gay, that makes their situation even harder.

they might make you break up. Maybe you also are afraid of losing your boyfriend or girlfriend. Maybe you think it's worth it to put up with anything just to have someone special in your life.

Every relationship has problems and upsets. That's just part of life. But if you see patterns of uncontrolled anger, jealousy, or possessiveness, or if there is shoving, slapping, forced sex, or other physical violence—even once—it's time to find help.

Think about this. Imagine that your best friend is going with someone who thinks and acts that way. Would it seem okay? Would you want them to stop hurting each other? Would you treat your best friend this way?

You have the right to be treated with respect and to not be harmed physically or emotionally by another person. Violence and abuse are not acceptable in any relationship. Love shouldn't hurt like this.

What's The First Step In Turning The Situation Around?

Take it seriously. Listen to yourself. If you feel that someone is abusing you, trust those feelings. Take it seriously.

What's The Second Step?

Take care of yourself. You're too valuable to settle for love that hurts. Don't stay silent—find support and help.

Why Does Violence Happen?

Often a relationship doesn't start out violent, but the violence starts after the two people have known each other for a while. The one big exception is forced sex (sometimes called "date rape" or "acquaintance rape"). Forced sex can sometimes happen the first or second time two people go out, especially when one person has very little dating experience and is afraid to say "no."

If you think something is wrong, it probably is. You may feel anxious, have trouble sleeping, or experience a change in appetite or weight. Your body may be telling you that something is not right—pay attention to these signs.

Violence is so common that sometimes it seems like the normal thing. But it's not. It's something we learn—and something we can change.

To understand why relationship violence happens, start by thinking about some of the situations you deal with every day.

Learning The Rules Of Love

When you first begin to go out with someone seriously, you have new and unfamiliar experiences. You start to discover society's rules for dating and relationship behavior. In addition, you are trying to figure out how to impress someone who is really special to you, and how to be yourself in a relationship. You see all kinds of images of what relationships are supposed to be like—but how do you know which ones are the right ones to follow? It's hard to ignore other people's examples of relationships—for example, if your mother and father don't show respect for each other. But you can decide for yourself what sort of relationships you want to have with your friends and your boyfriends or girlfriends. You can learn to have a healthy relationship and be loved and treated well by someone you care about. Violence is not the way to do it. Respect is.

Stereotypes That Hurt

In every culture, people have certain ideas about what it means to be a man or a woman. These ideas are called stereotypes. When you first start going out seriously, stereotypes can get you really confused about how you or the person you're going with ought to behave.

Boys often have the idea that it's a "guy thing" to act tough and to treat girls like property, like they own them. Guys often try to get their friends' approval by acting like they don't care about anything or anyone. Even a guy who likes a particular girl might show off for his friends by treating her badly or acting like she's been put on earth just to have sex with him.

Girls often accept the idea that it's a "guy thing" to push girls around, and so they should learn to go along with it. Girls also may believe it's a "girl thing" to try to figure out and do whatever will keep their boyfriends happy. So, they may feel they have to do only what the guy wants, or they may put up with the guy ignoring them, treating them badly around other guys, being really possessive, or being violent or abusive.

Both girls and boys often have the idea that boys can't control themselves when it comes to sex. They may believe that if a man forces a woman to have sex against her will, she was probably leading him on in some way.

Remember, there's no "guy thing" or "girl thing" when it comes to violence and abuse in relationships. There's just the "right thing" and the "wrong thing." Violence and abuse are always the wrong thing.

♣ It's A Fact!!

Violence is all around us— on television, in movies, in music videos, in computer games, and even in our schools, neighborhoods, and homes. People get into fights on the street, on buses, and in malls and use every kind of threat just to get their way. Drivers shout at and even shoot at each other. Television and movies show buildings and people being blown to bits. Bench-emptying brawls break out regularly on hockey, baseball, and football fields. Schools around the country use metal detectors and security guards to protect students from outsiders and from each other. And even at home, parents resort to violence to express their feelings to each other—and sometimes to their children.

Personal Pressures

Some social and personal situations are hard for anyone to handle, but they are especially hard when they affect teenagers. These personal pressures can contribute to abusive or violent behavior in relationships and to accepting that kind of behavior from a boyfriend or girlfriend.

Violence at home. When children see a parent being abused, they often grow up thinking that name-calling, screaming, or hitting is normal between people in love. Children in violent homes often get the idea that it is acceptable to threaten, intimidate, bully, or hit another person to get their own way.

Cultural beliefs. Teenagers' cultural and ethnic backgrounds affect their relationships. Some teenagers come from cultures in which people don't date someone unless they're going to marry that person, so they may not let their families know they are going out with someone. In some cultures, loyalty is such an important value that a teen in an abusive relationship may decide not to ask for help. Also, teenage girls who believe they can't do much with their lives because of their family's or culture's rules, or because of discrimination or poverty, may place their hopes for the future on finding someone to love and take care of them. Abuse may seem to them like a small price to pay to escape a life without hope.

Being lesbian, gay, or bisexual. Teenagers who are lesbian, gay, or bisexual face special pressures. When under a lot of stress from the outside world, some gay or lesbian teens may respond by getting angry at the person they're going out with. Even if victims decide they want help to stop the violence, they may not be able to get their friends, their teachers, or other adults to listen and understand what they're going through. If they haven't told anyone else about their sexual orientation, finding help also means taking the risk of coming out.

Having a disability. People who have disabilities often face a higher risk of violence of all kinds, especially if they are less able to defend themselves or to report abuse. Any behavior that intentionally harasses, teases, or takes advantage of a person with a disability is abusive. That includes such acts as keeping something out of reach of a person who uses a wheelchair, making it hard for someone who uses hearing aids to hear you, or deliberately trying to confuse someone with a learning disability.

Getting pregnant. Pregnancy is a vulnerable time that often leaves a teenage mother-to-be feeling alone, dependent, helpless, and condemned by parents, teachers, and friends. If her boyfriend is abusing her, she may not tell anyone because she fears losing him, doesn't want to face more disapproval from her family, or fears her baby will be taken away from her.

Drinking alcohol or taking drugs. Drinking alcohol or taking drugs does not cause violence, but it can have unpredictable effects: It can lower inhibitions or change perceptions of what is really going on. Even one drink is

♣ It's A Fact!!

If There's No Respect, It Isn't Love

Type of Violence	What It Means	How It Works	Early Warning Signs
Verbal Abuse	✔Behavior that causes harm with words	✔Name calling ✔Insults ✔Public humiliation ✔Yelling	✔Teasing that includes insults
Psychological and Emotional Abuse	✔Behavior intended to cause psychological or emotional distress	✔Threats, intimidation ✔Put-downs ✔Telling a person's secrets ✔Jealousy ✔Possessiveness ✔Isolating a person from friends, family ✔Destroying gifts, clothing, letters ✔Damaging a car, home, or other prized possessions	✔Pouting when you spend time with your friends ✔Threatening to leave you in an unsafe location ✔Trying to control what you do
Physical Abuse	✔Behaviors that inflict harm on a person	✔Slapping, hitting ✔Shoving, grabbing ✔Hair pulling, biting ✔Throwing objects at a person	✔Going into a rage when disappointed or frustrated ✔Teasing, tripping, or pushing ✔Threatening to injure
Sexual Violence: From Coercion to Date Rape	✔Sexual advances that make a person feel uncomfortable; sexual behavior that is unwanted	✔Insisting, physically or verbally, that a person who said "no" have sex anyway ✔Forced sex	✔Using emotional blackmail to talk you into having sex ("If you love me, you would...")
Abuse of Male Privilege: "It's a Guy Thing"	✔Behavior that assumes that boys have more power than girls and that boys have special privileges in relationships with girls	✔The guy makes all decisions for the couple ✔The guy expects his girlfriend to wait on and pamper him ✔The guy treats his girlfriend as if she is property he owns	✔Expecting you to be available to him at all times; he is available to you when he feels like it ✔Acting macho with friends: "This is my woman!"

enough for some teens to say or do things they regret. Alcohol and drugs also cause people to misread situations—to see a come-on when there isn't one, or to see only friendliness in a situation that could lead to rape or other violence. Drugs and alcohol often are used as excuses for abuse: "I didn't mean to hurt you. I was out of control." Being drunk or high is never an excuse for hurting someone.

Getting sexually involved with an adult. Young teenagers sometimes find themselves involved in sexual relationships with persons much older than they are. Although you may have romantic feelings for someone 5 or 10 years older, even if both of you consent to having sex, you should know that the older partner is committing a crime called statutory rape. Also, some adults beat or otherwise seek control over their young teen lovers. A sexual relationship where an adult dominates and controls a young teen should never be confused with love.

When You're Ready To Change The Situation

Hurting someone is never a sign of love. When a relationship is violent, the people involved need to either make the relationship work without violence or get out of it. You don't have to settle for an abusive relationship, and you don't have to continue to behave in abusive ways. Both of you deserve better.

People often need help to get out of abusive relationships. There are lots of reasons why breaking free can be hard.

- From a very early age, we get the idea that having a romantic relationship is the most important thing in the world and is worth any sacrifice.

- Going out with someone can be a status symbol, a way to feel more secure, or a way to break into a new circle of friends.

- Some people just don't like to be alone. They may feel that any relationship is better than no relationship.

- Many teenagers don't want to ask their parents for help. A girl whose boyfriend has slapped her might be afraid her parents won't let her go out with him or with anyone if they find out. A boy's parents might not approve of his girlfriend's influence and take away his car keys. The parents of a lesbian, gay, or bisexual teen might see one violent relationship as proof that all same-sex relationships are unhealthy.

Don't think the violence and abuse will just stop. Violent behavior won't disappear on its own. One or both of you may have wrong ideas about relationships, expressing anger, what to expect from each other, what you deserve from someone you love. Usually, both of you need support and help to make a change. Being hurt by someone that you care about can make you feel weak, worthless, helpless, and alone. Turning to drugs or alcohol is not a good way to handle the situation—it will not make the abuse disappear or feel more bearable.

Start by talking to someone. A counselor, a coach, a teacher, a parent, a doctor, a minister or rabbi, or a close friend can help you get an objective opinion of the situation. They may also have some good ideas to help you stop the hurting and start talking to each other about what you really want and need in a relationship.

If You Are The One Getting Hurt

If a person who claims to love you also threatens, intimidates, or injures you, that person has some wrong ideas about love and isn't worth your time. If you can't love someone without also feeling afraid of him or her, you're better off getting out of that relationship.

Assault is a crime. If you are afraid that someone you're going out with may hurt you badly, or if he or she already has, don't hesitate to call the police. In many states, teens who have been threatened or harmed can get the same restraining orders and other protections as adults.

The most important thing you can do is take care of yourself. As serious as the situation may seem, there are always alternatives to having a relationship with someone who hurts you. Demand to be treated with respect. You're worth it!

Make Sure You're Safe

Even if you haven't decided yet whether to leave the relationship, you can decide to be safe. Take some time to think about ways you can take yourself out of a dangerous situation the next time it occurs. For example, you can screen your phone calls, see your boyfriend or girlfriend only in a public place with other people around, or find a friend to stay with if you need to. Thinking through a plan of action can help you feel more in control of a situation so that you can take the next step.

Get Support

One of the most common forms of relationship violence is isolation—keeping you from spending time with your friends. If someone you're going out with controls your free time, you start to feel like you have nowhere else to turn. You aren't as likely to hear the support of friends who want you to leave the relationship. This is the time you need that support most. Talk to a friend, a teacher, a counselor, anyone who will support you as you stand up for yourself. Knowing that you don't have to rely only on yourself can give you the courage you need to break free. If the first person you talk to doesn't give you the support you need, try someone else. Don't give up!

Demand Respect

Point out the ways you've been hurt physically, sexually, and emotionally to the person you're going out with. Say that it's a big deal to you and that you want it to stop, now. This can be a hard step for many reasons. The person may deny the abuse, get furious and threaten to hurt you, your family, or himself or herself if you try to leave the relationship or tell anyone else about the problem. Or the person may get really sweet and remorseful, crying and promising never to hurt you again, only to return to the same old patterns later. Encourage the person you're going out with to find help in dealing with anger. Face facts, though: Most people won't make that change, even if they really love you. You can't change them. And as much as you might want to help the person you care about get over the abusive behavior, you have to think of yourself first.

Find Help

Just because this is your relationship doesn't mean you should try to solve the problem on your own. A boyfriend or girlfriend who is hurting you already doesn't respect you in the way you deserve. Talk to an adult—a teacher, coun-selor, coach, or friend—who will stick with you. Asking for help isn't a sign of weakness. It's about getting the support you deserve and making sure your boyfriend or girlfriend gets the message: Abuse is serious, and you deserve better.

If You Are The One Doing The Hurting

For your own sake and for the sake of the person you love, get help! The problem of hurting people when you're angry or frustrated or jealous is not going to go away on its own. Even if you honestly think you're some-times justified in your actions, you need to talk over this behavior with someone who can give you some new ideas about how to handle your feelings.

Drinking alcohol or using drugs does not make you hurt someone. It can have unpredictable effects, though, and can change the way you view situa-tions. You can never use drugs and alcohol as an excuse for abusive behavior. You should make it a reason to go for help for substance abuse.

Nobody is ever justified in hurting someone else to get their way. You're not going to get what you're looking for—love, respect, kindness, affection, a happy time with someone who loves and trusts you—unless you learn how to deal with your frustrations in a way that is not hurtful to others.

You're not a bad person—just someone who needs help to stop a bad behavior. You can learn new ways to deal with your anger, to fight fair, to communicate, and to give and get love in relationships. Don't let shame or fear stop you—talk to a parent, teacher, religious leader, doctor, nurse, psy-chologist, or guidance counselor today.

How Can I Help My Friend?

Seeing a friend in a violent relationship is painful. You might want to help but don't know what to say or do. You might be afraid of getting in-volved in someone else's problem. Or maybe you haven't seen the violence or abuse, and the person your friend is dating seems so nice that you wonder how much of the story to believe.

If You're Worried, Say Something

If you're concerned about your friend's safety, mention it. People who are being hurt in a relationship often feel they can't talk to anyone. They may be ashamed. They may think the abuse is their fault. They may think they deserve it. Let your friend know that you're there, you're willing to listen, and you're not going to judge. If your friend isn't ready to admit that there is a problem, don't give up. By being supportive and letting your friend know that someone is willing to listen, you're making it easier to start dealing with the problem.

Listen, Support, Believe

If a friend asks for your help, take it seriously. Believe what your friend tells you, not the gossip you might hear in the hallway. Your friend is trusting you with very personal and painful information—be a true friend and don't spread gossip. Give support by making it clear that your friend doesn't deserve to be abused in any way. Recognize that, as abusive as the person your friend is going out with might be, he or she may find it difficult to leave the relationship, particularly if your friend believes it will make the violence worse.

Help Your Friend Take Action

Help your friend develop a plan, whether it's telling the person to stop the abuse, confronting the person with other people, ending the relationship, or looking for help and safety. Help your friend practice what to say to the abusive person. Help your friend find and talk to a supportive adult, like a counselor. Find the phone number for a crisis center hotline in the yellow pages.

Call In Reinforcements

Your friend might tell you about a violent relationship only if you promise to keep it a secret. Violence and abuse are not problems to be kept secret. Whether your friend is ready to get help or not, find an adult you can talk to. Take your friend along if you can. You can tell the adult that you don't want to break a promise to keep a secret, but don't carry this burden all by yourself.

☞ Remember!!

Stopping violence in teen relationships is everyone's responsibility. Boyfriends, girlfriends, friends, parents, adults—all have a responsibility to speak out against behavior that is harmful and to prevent it from occurring.

Here are some people and organizations that can help. You can usually find phone numbers in your local phone book, or ask a counselor at school to help you get connected.

- State Domestic Violence Coalitions
- Local rape crisis centers
- Gay and lesbian resources/centers for teens
- 4H programs in rural areas
- Students Against Driving Drunk (SADD)
- National Domestic Violence Hotline, 1-800-799-SAFE
- National Organization for Victim Assistance, 1-800-TRY-NOVA
- National Resource Center on Domestic Violence, 1-800-537-2238
- Rape, Abuse, and Incest National Network, 1-800-656-HOPE
- Teachers, school counselors, school nurses
- Parents, pastors, neighbors, friends' parents
- Doctors and other health professionals
- Psychologists and other mental health professionals
- Police
- Shelters for battered women

Chapter 11

Physical And Emotional Abuse

Abuse Is A Big Problem

Child abuse is a big problem. In the United States, nearly 3 million children are reported as abused or neglected each year. Two thousand children are killed by child abuse each year. At least three children die each day from abuse.

Physical abuse is easy to describe. It can usually be recognized by the marks it leaves. Any beating, either by a hand or fist or with a weapon such as a belt or stick; any deliberate burning or other hurting of the skin; any neglect to properly feed or clothe a child may be called physical abuse.

Sometimes it is hard to decide if a child has been abused. Each family has different forms of discipline that may include physical punishment, such as spanking. But if spanking is used, it should never be so hard or so long that it leaves marks or injuries.

Emotional abuse is more difficult to describe and harder to recognize. Sometimes it involves things like the parent, step-parent or adult constantly calling the child names like "dummy" or "stupid." Or they may use obscene

About This Chapter: The text in this chapter is from " Physical and Emotional Abuse," produced by Children's Hospital for Teens, Akron, Ohio; reprinted with permission.

words, belittle the child, or tease him mercilessly. Emotional abuse leaves no marks—except on the child's spirit and self-esteem. The recognition of emotional abuse often requires the help of a trained professional.

Responding To Child Abuse

What can you do about child abuse if you or someone you know is experiencing it?

- *Get help to make a proper report.* If you are being abused, you may be afraid to tell anyone what is happening out of fear for what will happen to your caretaker. It is normal to be scared, but there are professionals in the community who can help you and your caretaker. Getting the assistance of a trained professional will help to protect you and get help for the adult who is doing the hurting as well. Reporting the abuse to your county child protective services, your local police department, or a counselor should initiate the help that your family needs.

- *Remember: You will be believed.* You may be afraid that no one will believe you if you tell about being hurt—especially if the hurt is emotional. People will believe you, but you must be prepared to tell your story several times. A counselor will help you know whom you should tell your story to. Physical abuse should first be reported to a medical person such as a school nurse, family doctor, or hospital. Emotional abuse needs to be evaluated by a trained counselor.

✎ Weird Words

Child Abuse: Causing physical, emotional, sexual, or psychological injury to a child, often by a parent, stepparent, or other caretaker. Child abuse may be the result of specific actions or the result of omissions of responsibility.

Child Neglect: The failure of a parent, stepparent, or responsible caretaker to provide for a child's physical, emotional, or nutritional needs.

- *Enter counseling.* Individual and family counseling can help you and your family cope with an abusive family member. Counseling can also help you to feel better about yourself and to identify ways to keep safe. Your school counselor, health care professional, or protective services worker can help you find the individual and family counseling services you need.

☞ Remember!!

Being abused is not a good way to grow up. But there is help for the child and the parent. If you are being abused or if you know someone who is, talk to your school nurse, counselor, family doctor, clergy person, or other trusted adult, or call your county child protective services or your local police department.

Chapter 12

The Impact Of Divorce On Teenagers

Mandy, now a sophomore in college, looks back on the time after her parents' divorce seven years ago, and recalls how much she hurt.

She remembers being told that, for children, the grief associated with their parents' divorce is nearly as great as that felt when a parent dies. Mandy thinks back to other emotions, too: anger, embarrassment, guilt, depression.

But now, she reminisces about a conversation that helped her feel better during one happy week of the troubled summer of her parents' separation. She and her sister were visiting their grandparents out of state, which was always a highlight of summer. That year it truly became a vacation away from the emotional atmosphere of their own home.

They weren't even talking about her parents' situation, but her grandfather was recalling his youth. His father had died of tuberculosis when he was 2 years old. Then in 1918, when he was only 7, his mother became critically ill during the massive flu epidemic that swept the country. He remembered feeling terribly frightened, with no father, a very sick mother, and a neighbor who took him and his brother into her home for six weeks. Happily, his mother recovered and was able to care lovingly for her sons until they left home as young adults.

About This Chapter: Text in this chapter is from "Divorce and the American Family," by Nancy Dreher, in *Current Health 2*, November 1996. © 1996 Weekly Reader Corporation; reprinted with permission.

✔ Quick Tip

Keeping A Family Strong In Times Of Conflict

What makes a strong family? Family Service America, an organization based in Milwaukee, Wisconsin, has identified these traits:

- appreciation for one another, in which parents and children treat each other with respect and listen to one another's opinions and feelings

- stable family rituals and sharing of stories of good times and bad times as a way of remembering and reaming

- seeking help when it's needed

- observing the strengths in other families, in a single-parent family, a family coping with problems, a family poorer than your own

Strength comes, too, from learning to handle conflicts. Family Service America points to these methods:

- taking a deep breath to resist reacting impulsively when you're upset

- awareness that everyone handles conflict differently

- weighing a conflict to determine if the issue is really a serious matter

- realizing what is truly at issue

- addressing a problem head-on, being specific and timely in confronting problems

- looking for areas of agreement

- exploring options

- giving one another credit for caring enough to make effort to address the matter that is causing the conflict

"You see," Mandy remembers him saying (and suddenly tied the dramatic events of his childhood to her own), "my mother, brother, and I had to cope with sad and difficult events, too. Divorce is sad and difficult, too, of course. But families have faced crises—different kinds of crises—all through history, and parents and children find ways to recover and move on. We were taken care of and you will be, too."

And those words, coming from her trusted grandfather, brought her comfort and helped her believe that things could begin to work out.

The Changing American Family

Divorce has changed the structure of the American family dramatically. Today it is estimated that five out of 10 first marriages will end in divorce. This means that a married couple is as likely to get a divorce as to stay married.

In 1960, the majority of families (53 percent) included a mother, father, and at least one child under 18, according to the U.S. Census Bureau. By 1995, only 36 percent of all families had this traditional form. The shape of families today is determined not only by divorce but by other factors as well. Far fewer parents of young children are lost to illness than when Mandy's grandfather was growing up. More than 30 percent of children born in America today are not part of a family with a mother and father married to one another.

What's Ideal?

At the same time, few people disagree that a child is best off living with both a mother and father. In an intact family, parents provide their children with day-to-day social and emotional support, offered from both a male and female adult perspective. In the majority of families today, a reliable financial base is provided by two working parents. Parents in a well-functioning marriage are role models who set an example for their children.

That's the ideal. And because it is, most people consider anything that deviates from it to be less than ideal. Because the benefits of a happy mom-dad-kids family are so obvious, being deprived of this scenario is what can make divorce so difficult, especially for the children involved. Even in a family where the pre-divorce atmosphere was extremely unpleasant, it's the sadness of what divorce represents that can bring grief to children—grief for the loss of a family they know they will no longer have.

Because divorce is so prevalent today, many families must find new ways to give the children of a divorce as many of the benefits of family life as possible. Even though the children no longer live with both Mom and Dad, they still can benefit from:

- a quality relationship with both parents (even if this is now on an individual basis) who can agree on priorities for their children

- financial support

- keeping a normal, active routine that allows them to pursue their own age-appropriate interests and friendships.

Confronting Emotions

Creating a new family arrangement after a divorce is not easily or quickly achieved. For both parents, going through the process of divorce involves complicated emotional, legal, and social issues that take their toll on both adults. Dealing with these issues sometimes even overshadows what should be so obvious—that their children's own emotions and needs require addressing as well. Tending to these emotions is the first step in arriving at a new sense of family.

One person who knows this so well is Suzy Yehl Marta, founder of an international organization called Rainbows that is headquartered in Illinois and offers a peer-support program for children who have experienced loss, principally through divorce. She recalls well-meaning people telling her at the time of her divorce more than 20 years ago: "Don't worry about your kids. They're resilient. They'll get over it."

Given the upheaval in her life at the time, she says, it would have been very convenient to believe that. But she sensed her children's pain. "When I was finally able to get them to talk about their feelings," she says, "their heartache was overwhelming."

How do you measure heartache? Kathryn Stich, an Atlanta, Georgia, school guidance counselor who leads support groups for children of divorce, cites these factors:

- Mood changes, swinging from relief (that their parents are no longer living together in a hostile atmosphere), resentment, and anger (that this has happened in the first place), guilt ("Was this my fault?"), and depression

- Overreaction, including a fear that life will never be normal again

- Loss of identity: Where do I belong if one of my parents has left? If we are no longer a family with a mom, dad, and kids, are we a family at all?

- Issues of custody: With whom will I live? When and how will I see my other parent? Who will support me?

- Concerns about parents: What about my parents' health—how will they hold up under the stress they're going through?

- Conflicts in loyalty: Can I be loyal to both my mom and dad? Will I be able to enjoy being with the parent I'm not living with? What will my relations be with all my grandparents, aunts, uncles, and cousins? How about my parents' friends?

- Taking on additional responsibilities at home: Will I have more work to do to help Mom (or Dad)? Will I need to get a job?

- Knowing where to turn: To whom can I turn to talk about my situation?

How can mood changes not be a part of a child's reaction to a divorce? Relief is probably the easiest emotion to accept. In the event of irreconcilable differences and a charged atmosphere between parents, separation and divorce can at least eliminate tension within the home. But there's also an opposing feeling that can almost be something like panic. Frustration with their parents' decision and fear about the future are common reactions.

Identity issues also are difficult to grapple with. Children usually align themselves with the parent who will have primary custody. This is especially

true if the divorce has been contentious or if the departing parent clearly
initiated the proceedings. But one of the clearest indicators of a healthy adjustment to divorce is a swift initiation of a consistent relationship with both
parents. Acceptance of the new situation is easier if both parents feel involved and responsible for their children, and if children see both parents
regularly and frequently.

In children, divorce can generate personal fears unrelated to their parents
or the security of their home environment: concern about how friends will
react to the news, fear of being embarrassed about the divorce, or even losing
popularity because of it.

✔ Quick Tip

"Find A Support Group."

That advice has helped many children of divorce. Being able to discuss your feelings with peers can take an enormous load off your mind.
Tremendous pressure can be relieved by talking over your emotions with
someone who has shared your experience, who doesn't know you or your
mom or dad, and who won't talk about what's been said once he or she
leaves the room.

Rainbows, a not-for-profit organization based in Schaumburg, Illinois, has provided support to more than 600,000 children, teens, and
adults who are grieving over a death, divorce, or other painful transition
in the family. For more information, call 800-266-3206.

Another organization with resources for children going through divorce is Family Service America, Inc., which offers free information and
referral to local family service agencies all around the country. The organization can be reached at 800-221-2681.

Setting The Tone For The New Family

Working out custody for the children can be one of the most complicated issues in a divorce, involving both legal and physical custody. Some types of custody arrangements include:

- In joint legal custody, both parents are considered equal partners in raising their children and equally involved in major decisions relating to them. Joint legal custody is not related to the amount of time children spend with one parent or another. Joint physical custody, on the other hand, may mean that children spend an equal amount of time with each parent, or certain specific times of the year with each parent.

- With sole legal custody, one parent alone has legal control over all decisions relating to the children. The noncustodial parent has no legal rights relating to the children, except a legally defined time of access to them.

Custody decisions set the tone for the new family unit. The arrangements made will define where the child will live, how often and how much time the children will spend with the parent who doesn't live in the home anymore, and how the children will be supported.

The Money Issue

Financial support plays a critical and complicated role in the establishment of the new family unit. At the time of a divorce, a couple has to address questions of division of property (home and possessions), assets (money in bank accounts, for example), and debts (a mortgage on a house, for example).

Child support is a crucial part of this. Child support is money paid by the noncustodial to the custodial parent for the children's day-to-day expenses. The amount depends on the income of both parents, and can change if new circumstances arise, such as a remarriage or a significant change in income of one parent. The payments usually continue until a child reaches a certain age or marries or finds full-time employment.

Seen individually, secure financial arrangements can contribute to a healthy adjustment to divorce—or deprive children of basic necessities. Failure to pay child support has become a national issue.

In many cases, financial restraints in general mean that most parents need to adjust their lifestyle. A divorce, for example, involves setting up two households where there used to be one. If money is tight, certain activities or expenses that used to be easily covered can become less affordable.

Can I Still Love Mom and Dad?

Conflicts in loyalty present some of the thorniest issues for children of divorce. It's ideal for both parents to show a sense of responsibility and respect for one another after a divorce, making it easier for children to love and enjoy the company of both parents. But often the conflicts that accompany a divorce leave parents angry and resentful about their divorced partner and very vocal about him or her, even in front of the children. As a result, kids can be caught in the crossfire and faced with a dilemma: Can I still love Dad even if Mom says he's unfair or cruel or just plain wrong about things?

Some divorced parents try to influence their children to take sides and use a child's expressed loyalty to hurt the divorced spouse. Kids can be very confused if they are put under pressure to take sides. Often, they can grow up with strong feelings of resentment toward both their mother and their father.

Relatives are another issue. The definition of family includes not only parents and children, but in most cases, a wider circle of relatives who are often very important in the lives of children. Grandparents, aunts and uncles, and cousins are a part of the family associated with good times and happy rituals. At the time of a divorce, grandparents (remember Mandy's?) can have a stabilizing effect on children, providing them with a sense of continuity among the three generations of the family.

This is why experts feel it is best when children remain in contact with both sets of grandparents and with other close relatives. Even if relations are strained by the divorce (and often complicated by distance), keeping up at times of birthdays and other holidays can preserve important links.

The Home Front

No doubt a child's immediate world—the world at home—hangs in different ways when parents divorce and one parent moves out. Many children are required to take on additional responsibilities for chores, babysitting, even attending events in the place of the absent parent. Some parents begin to relate to their child as a mini-adult, sharing confidences and becoming emotionally dependent on the children. This may contribute to a child's developing maturity, but it also has risks. Children need same-age friends and confidants. They also need to be able to pursue activities and someday leave home without feeling guilty because they are leaving an emotionally needy parent.

Many children of divorce—especially teens—say they are helped by the realization that after all is said and done, they must get on with their own life.

Says Dr. Mark Singer, who has counseled families and children for 22 years: "By developing their own interests and skills, children can nurture their own sense of self. Putting forth an effort to learn a new sport, for example, or an activity they can call their own can make them less dependent on others. They can see that life goes on. They'll be OK."

☞ Remember!!

Counselors who have worked with children of divorce say that many young people come through the experience as stronger, more mature individuals. Many find they consciously build better relationships with both parents and even their own friends. They grow into adulthood having learned a lot about life and relationships, what doesn't work...and what does.

Chapter 13

Teens And Grief

Unfortunately, the needs of the bereaved teenager have been sorely overlooked for decades. In many grief recovery programs, support is often available for younger children and adults, but there is a definite void in teen services. I have seen this void throughout our country. Teenagers often give us mixed messages. They tell us that they need and expect our help in providing them with food and a nurturing environment but also tell us, on the other hand, that they can run their lives on their own. Because people do not always know how to respond to teens, they frequently back off, resulting in a teen who is left to grieve alone or with very limited support.

What Makes Adolescent Grief Different From That Experienced By An Adult?

Adolescence is perhaps one of the most difficult and confusing stages in life. It is a time of change and with every change, comes a grieving process. As an example:

- The teenager who has a brother or sister move out of the house to get married or go to school will have to adjust to life in the home without their sibling. Meals and family events will not be spent together with the frequency of the past.

About This Chapter: Text in this chapter is from "Grief and the Adolescent," by Linda Cunningham, © 1996 Teen Age Grief, Inc. (TAG); reprinted with permission.

- Divorce in a family will also bring about a grieving process as one parent leaves the home.

- Children who have been abused or sexually molested will experience the loss of innocence and control of their bodies—a very painful grieving process.

- The dating process, a very natural process in adolescence, also involves grief as relationships build and then dissolve as they discover who they are and what they want in life.

- Death of a pet. A pet is one of the few sources of unconditional love that life affords us. We can tell a pet our secrets, and in most cases, the pet is always glad to see us. Losing a pet can bring about profound grief in many children and adults alike.

> ✎ **Weird Words**
>
> Bereavement: A normal, intense state of suffering and sadness after a loss, such as the death of a loved one.
>
> Chronic Grief: Unresolved grief accompanied with denial of loss.
>
> Dysfunctional Grief: Protracted grief following unsuccessful attempts to work through emotional issues related to loss.
>
> Grief Reaction: An intense emotional response to a profound loss, such as the death of a loved one or the loss of something valued, symptoms can include fatigue, emptiness, hyperventilation, diminished interest in eating, and insomnia.

- Abortion: Whether we are in agreement or disagreement with the issues of abortion, when it occurs, there is a very real loss that is experienced both by the mother and father. This loss frequently comes back to the surface as other pregnancies occur later on in life.

These are only a few of the grief issues that a teen may experience as a natural part of growing up. Add to these experiences the death of a loved one, and you are likely to find a child who is terribly confused and in great pain.

Experiences Of The Bereaved Teenager

Because grief can be very complex and unique to every individual, we will address the more frequent reactions of teenagers who are grieving.

Shock/Disbelief

Knowing, intellectually, that someone has died does not always mean that the death seems real, especially in the early days and weeks of bereavement. Many teens experience what I call "automatic pilot": they function as usual but with a feeling that "this really didn't happen." Teenagers, in particular, may show little signs of grieving in the beginning. This numbness or form of denial is an important coping mechanism and should be respected. In months to come, the numbness will fade and they will need you more than ever. If the teenager witnesses a traumatic death, this state of shock and disbelief could last for months. Be prepared for signs of post-traumatic stress such as flashbacks, nightmares, etc.

Guilt

Most people who grieve experience some level of guilt. We put ourselves through the "If onlys": If only I could have prevented the death; If only I hadn't had that argument; If only I had said "I love you." Arguments are a part of family life, especially during adolescence. Because of this fact, teenagers often experience extreme feelings of guilt or take on responsibility for the death in some way. It is important that we do not try to "fix" their grief. Most teens simply need to tell you what they are feeling and, in time, the guilt, with good support, can diminish.

Unusual Happenings

It is not at all uncommon for a bereaved teenager to hear the voice of the deceased or feel as though they see that person passing by or in a crowd. These occurrences can be frightening unless there is someone around to let them know that this is a natural part of the grieving process.

Thoughts Of Suicide

It is not uncommon for a teenager to have thoughts of suicide as a way of escaping pain or joining their loved one. It is important that these thoughts can be shared in a safe environment without the fear of judgment or panic from the person who is listening. Wanting to escape the pain is a normal response. When teens are made aware of the fact that these thoughts often accompany grief, that in itself can offer some relief. This subject should always be handled with great care. If the teenager is describing to you a method of how they plan to take their life, this is clearly a "red flag" and professional help should be made available immediately.

Sexual Activity

It is not unusual for a teenager to become sexually active during the grief process. If the teen has lost a family member, frequently other family members will not be available for them emotionally, because they, too, are in pain. The need to be close to someone, both physically and emotionally, can be very strong at this time and sexual activity can also serve as a distraction from their pain.

Drugs/Alcohol

When teens are grieving, it is a very natural response to want to numb the pain—when someone is drunk or high, they do not have to feel. Bereaved teens are at high risk for involving themselves in self-destructive behavior. While these drugs may temporarily numb the pain, they very clearly prolong and complicate the grieving process. It is important to be open with the teenager in this area without pointing a judgmental finger.

Anger

When we have been abandoned through death, anger can become very powerful. Many teens have said "I want to punch someone out" or "I want to destroy something." It is important that teens be given healthy options in expressing their anger. Some suggestions might include: screaming into a pillow;

> ## ❖ It's A Fact!!
>
> People cope with grief in many different ways. The grief process can include:
>
> - Shock and disbelief
> - Guilt
> - Seeing or hearing a deceased loved one
> - Suicidal thoughts
> - Sexual activity
> - Alcohol or other drug use
> - Anger
> - Tears

pounding a mattress; ripping Kleenex out of a box until it is empty; throwing ice cubes at a wall or nearby tree. All of these expressions of anger release the physical energy that words alone cannot. It is important to note, also, that none of these expressions of anger will hurt the teenager or those around him or her.

Tears

Tears are a natural and necessary part of grief. If you do not see the tears, do not assume they are not there. Many teens will grieve privately, crying in the shower, in their rooms or alone at the gravesite. If a teenager should share his or her tears with you, be still, be quiet and listen—don't try to fix their pain.

How Can You Help?

Every teenager needs to grieve in their own time and in their own way. To try and speed up the recovery process could be harmful. Listed below are some suggestions for helping the bereaved teenager.

- Ask to see a picture of the person who has died. Let them tell you about this person and why they were special. Have them share some special memories with you.

- Let the teenager tell you about their experience with the death; where they were when the death occurred, what happened immediately afterwards and what are they experiencing right now. Adults who avoid the subject or put on a front may create an atmosphere of isolation and confusion. The teenager may assume others really didn't love the deceased. They may also assume, because others do not appear to be grieving, that there must be something wrong with them—this can be very frightening.

- Let the teen tell you about any dreams they have had regarding the death of their loved one. Dreams can be very powerful and a listening ear can provide needed support.

- Writing a letter to the deceased can often provide an opportunity for the teenager to say good-bye to their loved one. While this can be a painful exercise, it frequently provides relief and a safe expression of feelings. Writing a letter to someone they love who is still alive can also be helpful. Many times teens will distance themselves from loved ones fearing that they could lose again and it would be more pain than they could bare. This letter can help them to reconnect with the important people in their lives.

- Making a collage can be a creative way of enhancing the healing process in grief. Let the teenager gather magazines and cut out words and pictures that remind them of the deceased and place them on construction paper. When they complete this project, they will find that they have told a story through their collage. These collages become treasured items. Frequently they are placed in a visible place in the home where people visiting will ask questions about it, affording the teen the opportunity to talk about their loved one without having to bring up the subject themselves.

- Help the teenager identify what they need during this time and encourage them to let others know what they need. The common complaint of many bereaved is that people don't seem to care and they are not around when you need them. Frequently people are not around because they don't know what to do or say and they back off for fear of creating more pain. If we don't tell people what we need, we remain a victim and victims seldom heal.

> ☞ **Remember!!**
>
> Your presence and the expression of genuine support will be a gift grieving teens can carry with them for a lifetime. For more information about adolescent grief, contact:
>
> **TAG: Teen Age Grief, Inc.**
> P.O. Box 220034
> Newhall, CA 91322-0034
> Phone: 661-253-1932
> Fax: 661-245-2536
> Website: http://www.smartlink.net/~tag
> E-Mail: tag@thevine.net

Chapter 14

When Your Parent Has A Mental Illness

Growing up in any family can be challenging at times, but there are often special problems and challenges for families in which one or both parents have a mental illness. Children in these families often have to deal with instability or unpredictability. Often there is confusion in family roles and children have to take over many of the adult responsibilities, such as taking care of younger brothers and sisters or managing household duties normally managed by adults. They may even have the responsibility of taking care of the emotional or physical needs of their parents.

Children in these situations do not always receive the parental care and nurturing they need. Often they feel ashamed to talk about their situation with others and consequently may withdraw from relatives or friends who could help them or support them. Often unable to articulate their needs, even to themselves, these children frequently feel isolated and alone.

Children of mentally ill parents may also experience added difficulties as adults. These may include:

- **Relationship difficulties:**
  - difficulty in initiating relationships, and experiencing feelings of isolation

About This Chapter: Text in this chapter is from "When Your Parent Has A Mental Illness," a brochure developed by Counseling Center at the University of Illinois at Urbana-Champaign, © 1996 by The Board of Trustees of the University of Illinois; reprinted with permission.

- difficulty in romantic relationships
- difficulty in maintaining friendships
- difficulty with trusting self and others
- difficulty balancing level of intimacy (excessive dependence or excessive avoidance)
- difficulty balancing taking care of self and taking care of others

- **Emotional difficulties:**
  - guilt, resentment
  - shame, embarrassment
  - depression
  - fear of inheriting parent's mental illness
  - fear of discovery by partner, friends
  - inability to express anger constructively, angry outbursts or repressed anger
  - confusion about one's own identity
  - negative outlook on life
  - inability to deal with life unless it is chaotic or in crisis
  - overly responsible or irresponsible in many areas of life such as commitments, money, alcohol, relationships, etc.
  - self defeating thoughts, attitudes, and behaviors such as "I don't matter; I'm not worth much; It's no use trying."
  - self defeating themes involving a tendency to equate achievement with worth as a person, such as: "Maybe I can matter if I can excel at something, be perfect in school, my job, my relationships. But if I fail, I'm worthless and it's terrible."

If you are experiencing any of these difficulties, you are not alone. It is helpful to recognize that these problematic feelings and behaviors helped you to cope and survive the more vulnerable years of childhood. Your recognition that they limit your life choices as an adult is the beginning of your search for more rewarding and functional ways of relating.

How You Can Help Yourself

1. Acknowledge that you have a parent with a mental illness and acknowledge the effects this has had on you.

    *   acknowledge previously inadmissible feelings such as anger, shame, guilt, etc.

    *   grieve the parental support you never received.

    *   remember that you are not responsible for causing your parent's problems or for fixing his/her condition.

2. Develop new ways of taking care of yourself.

    *   recognize your own legitimate needs and begin taking care of them

    *   recognize the stressors in your life, and learn ways of managing them.

    *   replace negative thoughts with more positive statements: "I am a worthwhile person. This truth does not depend on my successes or failures. My life has ups and downs, but my worth does not change."

✔ Quick Tip

The Counseling Center at the University of Illinois at Urbana-Champaign suggests these books as additional sources of information:

*   Diner, Sherry H. *Nothing to Be Ashamed of: Growing up with Mental Illness in Your Family.* New York: Lothrop, Lee & Shepard Books, 1989.

*   Duke, Patty. *A Brilliant Madness: Living with Manic-Depressive Illness.* New York: Bantam Books, 1992.

*   Forward, Susan. *Toxic Parents.* New York: Bantam Books, 1990.

*   Greenberg, Harvey R. *Emotional Illness in Your Family: Helping Your Relative, Helping Yourself.* New York: Macmillan, 1989.

*   Walsh, Maryellen. *Schizophrenia: Straight Talk for Family and Friends.* New York: Morrow, 1985.

3. Develop new ways of relating to others.

   - recognize old unhealthy family patterns of communicating, and practice new ways of relating to parents and other family members.

   - recognize the difficulties you have with relationships, and learn new ways of relating to others.

   - appreciate and enjoy stability in your relationships, recognizing that relationships don't have to be defined by crisis or dependency.

4. Explore other resources.

Educate Yourself About Your Parent's Illness

This can help you understand what your parent is facing and what has caused problems for your family. It can also aid in relieving your feelings of guilt, resentment, embarrassment, and shame.

Consider Seeing A Mental Health Professional

A counselor can help you understand how your parent's illness impacts your life. Also a counselor can help you learn healthier ways of relating to others and caring for your own needs.

Join A Support Group

A support group that addresses your specific situation can help reduce feelings of isolation. Seeking such support can be especially helpful when family members are either uncomfortable with or refuse to acknowledge the problem.

Chapter 15

Information For Brothers And Sisters Of People With Mental Disorders

Common Concerns And Reactions Of Siblings

Following are some of the things the sibling (brother or sister) of someone with mental illness may be thinking. By understanding these thoughts, you will be better able to deal with them.

- Siblings of the mentally ill person are profoundly affected emotionally in relationships with families and friends, and thoughts of own self image.

- He/she may try to escape, physically and/or emotionally from the family. May establish rigid boundaries/barriers to separate self from others.

- The healthy sibling may take sides with one or both parents or with the ill sibling or with other siblings. He/she may try to act as a mediator, and may have conflicting feelings of feeling sorry for, and angry with parents and the ill sibling.

- Healthy sibling may feel need to make up for ill sibling's failings or to avoid creating more problems.

About This Chapter: This chapter contains information from "Information for Brothers and Sisters of People with Neurobiological Disorders" which was excerpted from http://www.schizophrenia.com/ami/coping/brosis.html, © by NAMI (National Alliance for the Mentally Ill). Reprinted with permission of the National Alliance for the Mentally Ill. Additional reading list updated by the editor in 2001.

- May feel parents give all attention to the ill kid.

- May feel more "serious" about life. Atmosphere at home may be more serious, intense.

- May feel concerned about how to respond effectively during a crisis with the ill family member.

- The healthy sibling may establish a more critical, realistic view of parents earlier—also may become closer to parents.

- The healthy sibling may be concerned about who will take care of the ill sibling when the parents no longer can. Should I?

- Concerns about whether he/she too could be or become mentally ill.

- Concerns about whether or not to have kids.

- May work hard to prove to others that they are "different" from sibling (not ill).

- Guilt—because of anger. Resentment—because one is not ill, over one's advantages, over one's treatment of ill sibling—did I contribute to the problem?

- Stigma/embarrassment over person's behavior and reaction of general public who know little about mental illness—resulting in isolation.

- Grief because of loss of brother or sister as once knew him or her.

- Difficulty establishing relationship with sibling.

- Disagreement with diagnosis, treatment, and frustration at not having any real power to impact.

- Confusion about causes of illness—Environmental? Chemical? Hereditary?

What Your Parents Can't Do

- Can't take away fact that the mental illness impacts on other siblings.

- Can't lessen the impact by not talking about it.

- Can't shield the siblings from their own feelings about it.

- Can't determine the individual coping style siblings may adopt.

- Can't do the grieving (mourning) process for you. This involves denial, sadness, anger, and finally, acceptance. This process everyone must do in an individual way at an individual pace.

- Can't make you seek help if you need the denial stage.

- Can't take away peer and societal stigma.

What Your Parents Can Do

- Be aware that all family members are profoundly affected.

- Be aware of the coping stance the siblings adopt; for example, estrangement, enmeshment, etc.

- Talk about feelings and encourage you to do the same.

- Learn about the illness to lower family anxiety.

- Do not make the ill member the axis in which the family revolves. This is as detrimental to the ill person as it is to the other family members.

- Seek to improve the mental health system so that after-care options are available.

- Encourage you to join a support group specifically for siblings and adult children of the mentally ill.

Additional Reading

The following books may be available at your school or local public library or from a bookstore:

- *Siblings of the Mentally Ill*, by Wendy Carlisle; R&E Publishers, 1984. (ISBN: 0882477056)

- *Hidden Victims—Hidden Healers: An Eight Stage Healing Process for Family and Friends of the Mentally Ill*, by Julie T. Johnson; PEMA Publications, Inc., 1994. (ISBN: 0964043009)

- *Troubled Journey: Coming to Terms with the Mental Illness of a Sibling or Parent*, by Diane T. Marsh and Rex M. Dickens; Putnam, 1997. (ISBN: 0874778751)

- *How to Cope with Mental Illness in Your Family: A Self-Care Guide for Siblings, Offspring, and Parents*, by Diane T. Marsh, Rex M. Dickens, and E. Fuller Torrey; J.P. Tarcher, 1998. (ISBN: 0874779235)

- *My Sister's Keeper: Learning to Cope with a Sibling's Mental Illness*, by Margaret Moorman; Viking Penguin USA, 1993. (ISBN: 0140231218)

- *When Madness Comes Home: Help and Hope for the Children, Siblings, and Partners of the Mentally Ill*, by Victoria Secunda; Hyperion, 1998. (ISBN: 078688326X)

- *Mad House: Growing Up in the Shadow of Mentally Ill Siblings*, by Clea Simon; Penguin USA, 1998. (ISBN: 0140274340)

- *When Someone You Love Has a Mental Illness: A Handbook for Family, Friends, and Caregivers*, by Rebecca Woolis and Agnes Hatfield; J.P. Tarcher, 1992. (ISBN: 0874776953)

Part 2

Common Types Of Mental Illness

Chapter 16

Mental, Emotional, And Behavior Disorders: An Overview

Young people can have mental, emotional, and behavior problems that are real, painful, and costly. These problems, often called "disorders," are a source of stress for the child as well as the family, school, community, and larger society.

The number of families who are affected by mental, emotional, and behavior disorders in young people is staggering. It is estimated that as many as one in five children or adolescents may have a mental health problem that can be identified and treated. At least 1 in 10—or as many as 6 million young people—may have a "serious emotional disturbance." This term refers to a mental health problem that severely disrupts a person's ability to function socially, academically, and emotionally.

Mental health disorders in children and adolescents are caused by biology, environment, or a mix of both. Examples of biological factors are genetics, chemical imbalances in the body, and damage to the central nervous system, such as a head injury. Many factors in a young person's environment can affect his or her mental health, such as exposure to violence, extreme stress, and loss of an important person.

About This Chapter: Text is this chapter is taken from " Mental, Emotional, and Behavior Disorders in Children and Adolescents," a fact sheet produced by the Center for Mental Health Services (CMHS), a federal agency within the U.S. Department of Health and Human Services, December 1998.

Caring families and communities working together can help children and adolescents with mental disorders. A broad range of services often is necessary to meet the needs of these young people and families.

The Disorders

Following are descriptions of some of the mental, emotional, and behavior problems that can occur during childhood and adolescence. All of these disorders can have a serious impact on a child's overall health. Some disorders are more common than others, and conditions can range from mild to severe. Often, a child has more than one disorder. This chapter contains estimates of the prevalence (number of existing cases in a defined time period) of mental, emotional, and behavior disorders. These estimates are taken from several sources, most of which are small-scale studies that can yield only a rough gauge of prevalence rates. The National Institute of Mental Health is currently engaged in a nationwide study to determine with greater accuracy the prevalence of mental disorders among children and adolescents. This information is needed to increase understanding of mental health problems and to improve the treatment and services that help young people who are affected by these conditions.

♣ **It's A Fact!!**

In this chapter, "**Mental Health Problems**" for children and adolescents refers to the range of all diagnosable emotional, behavioral, and mental disorders. They include depression, attention-deficit/hyperactivity disorder, and anxiety, conduct, and eating disorders. Mental health problems affect one in every five young people at any given time.

"**Serious Emotional Disturbances**" for children and adolescents refers to the above disorders when they severely disrupt daily functioning in home, school, or community. Serious emotional disturbances affect 1 in every 10 young people at any given time.

Source: "Prevalence of serious emotional disturbance in children and adolescents," Mental Health, United States, 1996. *Center for Mental Health Services, Substance Abuse and Mental Health Services Administration, U.S. Department of Health and Human Services, 1996.*

Anxiety Disorders

Anxiety disorders are the most common of the childhood disorders. They affect an estimated 8 to 10 of every 100 children and adolescents. These young people experience excessive fear, worry, or uneasiness that interferes with their daily lives. Anxiety disorders include:

- *Phobia:* An unrealistic and overwhelming fear of some object or situation;

- *Generalized Anxiety Disorder:* A pattern of excessive, unrealistic worry not attributable to any recent experience;

- *Panic Disorder:* Terrifying panic attacks that include physical symptoms such as rapid heartbeat and dizziness;

- *Obsessive-Compulsive Disorder:* Being trapped in a pattern of repeated thoughts and behaviors such as counting or handwashing; and

- *Post-Traumatic Stress Disorder:* A pattern of flashbacks and other symptoms that occurs in children who have experienced a psychologically distressing event such as physical or sexual abuse, being a victim or witness of violence, or exposure to some other traumatic event such as a bombing or hurricane.

Mood Disorders

Major depression is recognized more and more in young people. Years ago, many people believed that major depression did not occur in childhood. But we now know that the disorder can occur at any age. Studies show that up to 6 out of every 100 children may have depression. The disorder is marked by changes in:

- *Emotion:* The child often feels sad, cries, looks tearful, feels worthless;

- *Motivation:* Schoolwork declines, the child shows no interest in play;

- *Physical Well-Being:* There may be changes in appetite or sleep patterns and vague physical complaints; and

- *Thoughts:* The child believes that he or she is ugly, that he or she is unable to do anything right, or that the world or life is hopeless.

Some adolescents or even elementary school children with depression may not place any value on their own lives, which may lead to suicide.

Bipolar disorder (manic-depressive illness) in children and adolescents is marked by exaggerated mood swings between extreme lows (depression) and highs (excitedness or manic phases). Periods of moderate mood occur in between. During a manic phase, the child or adolescent may talk nonstop, need very little sleep, and show unusually poor judgment. Bipolar mood swings can recur throughout life.

❖ **It's A Fact!!**

Adults with bipolar disorder (which is as common as 1 in 100 adults) often experienced their first symptoms during their teenage years.

Other Common Disorders

Attention-deficit/hyperactivity disorder occurs in up to 5 of every 100 children. A young person with attention-deficit/hyperactivity disorder is unable to focus attention and is often impulsive and easily distracted. Most children with this disorder have great difficulty remaining still, taking turns, and keeping quiet. Symptoms must be evident in at least two settings (for instance, at home and at school) for attention-deficit/hyperactivity disorder to be diagnosed.

Learning disorders affect the ability of children and adolescents to receive or express information. These problems can show up as difficulties with spoken and written language, coordination, attention, or self-control. Such difficulties can make it harder for a child to learn to read, write, or do math. Approximately 5 of every 100 children in public schools are identified as having a learning disorder.

Conduct disorder causes children and adolescents to act out their feelings or impulses toward others in destructive ways. Young people with conduct disorder repeatedly violate the basic rights of others and the rules of society. The offenses that these children and adolescents commit often get more serious over time. Examples include lying, theft, aggression, truancy, firesetting, and vandalism. Children and adolescents with conduct disorder usually have little care or concern for others. Current research has yielded varying estimates of the number of young people with this disorder; most estimates range from 4 to 10 of every 100 children and adolescents.

Eating disorders can be life threatening. A young person with anorexia nervosa, for example, cannot be persuaded to maintain a minimally normal body weight. This child or adolescent is intensely afraid of gaining weight and doesn't believe that he or she is underweight. Anorexia affects 1 in every 100 to 200 adolescent girls and a much smaller number of boys.

Youngsters with bulimia nervosa feel compelled to binge (eat huge amounts of food at a time). Afterward, to prevent weight gain, they rid their bodies of the food by vomiting, abusing laxatives, taking enemas, or exercising obsessively. Reported rates vary from 1 to 3 out of 100 young people.

Autism spectrum disorder or **autism** appears before a child's third birthday. Children with autism have problems interacting and communicating with others. They behave inappropriately, often repeating behaviors over long periods. For example, some children bang their heads, rock, or spin objects. The impairments range from mild to severe. Children with autistic disorder may have a very limited awareness of others and are at increased risk for other mental disorders. Studies suggest that autism spectrum disorder affects 7 to 14 of every 10,000 children.

Schizophrenia can be a devastating mental disorder. Young people with schizophrenia have psychotic periods when they may have hallucinations (sense things that do not exist, such as hearing voices), withdraw from others, and lose contact with reality. Other symptoms include delusional or disordered thoughts and an inability to experience pleasure. Schizophrenia is even more rare than autism in children under 12, but occurs in about 3 out of every 1000 adolescents.

Treatment, Support Services, And Research: Sources Of Hope

Many of the symptoms and much of the distress associated with childhood and adolescent mental, emotional, and behavior problems may be alleviated with timely and appropriate treatment and support services.

A child or adolescent in need of treatment or services and his or her family may need a plan of care based on the severity and duration of symptoms. Optimally, this plan is developed with the family, service providers, and a service coordinator, who is referred to as a case manager. Whenever possible, the child or adolescent is involved in decisions.

Tying together all the various supports and services in a plan of care for a particular child and family is commonly referred to as a "system of care." A system of care is designed to improve the child's ability to function in all areas of life—at home, at school, and in the community. For a fact sheet on systems of care, call the Center for Mental Health Services at 1-800-789-2647.

> **✔ Quick Tip**
>
> In a "System of Care," local organizations work in teams—with families as critical partners—to provide a full range of services to children and adolescents with serious emotional disturbances. The team strives to meet the unique needs of each young person and his or her family in or near their home. These services should also address and respect the culture and ethnicity of the people they serve. (For more information on systems of care, call the Center for Mental Health Services at 1-800-789-2647).

Researchers are working to produce new knowledge and understanding about mental, emotional, and behavior disorders. Studies are also exploring ways to prevent and treat mental, emotional, and behavior problems, including the range of services that may be required.

Many of these studies are funded by Federal agencies within the Department of Health and Human Services, which include:

- the National Institutes of Health
- the National Institute of Mental Health
- the National Institute of Child Health and Human Development
- the National Institute for Drug Abuse
- the National Institute on Alcoholism and Alcohol Abuse
- the Substance Abuse and Mental Health Services Administration
- the Center for Mental Health Services
- the Center for Substance Abuse Prevention
- the Center for Substance Abuse Treatment
- the Administration for Children and Families
- the Health Resources and Services Administration

Related activities are taking place within:

- the Department of Education
- the Department of Justice

There is now more reason than ever for youngsters with these problems and their families to lead normal, happy lives.

☞ Remember!!

- Every child's mental health is important.
- Many children have mental health problems.
- These problems are real and painful and can be severe.
- Mental health problems can be recognized and treated.
- Caring families and communities working together can help.
- Information is available; call the Center for Mental Health Services at 1-800-789-2647 (TTY: 301-443-9006).

Chapter 17

Dealing With The Depths Of Depression

Imagine attending a party with these prominent guests: Abraham Lincoln, Theodore Roosevelt, Robert Schumann, Ludwig Von Beethoven, Edgar Allen Poe, Mark Twain, Vincent Van Gogh, and Georgia O'Keefe. Maybe Schumann and Beethoven are at the dinner table intently discussing the crescendos in their most recent scores, while Twain sits on a couch telling Poe about the plot of his latest novel. O'Keefe and Van Gogh may be talking about their art, while Roosevelt and Lincoln discuss political endeavors.

But in fact, these historical figures also had a much more personal common experience: Each of them battled the debilitating illness of depression.

It is common for people to speak of how "depressed" they are. However, the occasional sadness everyone feels due to life's disappointments is very different from the serious illness caused by a brain disorder. Depression profoundly impairs the ability to function in everyday situations by affecting moods, thoughts, behaviors, and physical well-being.

Twenty-seven-year-old Anne (not her real name) has suffered from depression for more than 10 years. "For me it's feelings of worthlessness," she explains. "Feeling like I haven't accomplished the things that I want to or

About This Chapter: Text in this chapter is from "Dealing with the Depths of Depression," by Liora Nordenberg in *FDA Consumer*, U.S. Food and Drug Administration, July/August 1998.

feel I should have and yet I don't have the energy to do them. It's feeling disconnected from people in my life, even friends and family who care about me. It's not wanting to get out of bed some mornings and losing hope that life will ever get better."

Depression strikes about 17 million American adults each year—more than cancer, AIDS, or coronary heart disease—according to the National Institute of Mental Health (NIMH). An estimated 15 percent of chronic depression cases end in suicide. Women are twice as likely as men to be affected.

❖ **It's A Fact!!**

According to the U.S. Department of Health and Human Services, major depression affects 15 percent of Americans at one point during their lives. Despite this high prevalence, the National Alliance for the Mentally Ill estimates that it takes an average of eight years from the onset of depression to get a proper diagnosis.

Many people simply don't know what depression is. "A lot of people still believe that depression is a character flaw or caused by bad parenting," says Mary Rappaport, a spokeswoman for the National Alliance for the Mentally Ill. She explains that depression cannot be overcome by willpower, but requires medical attention.

Fortunately, depression is treatable, says Thomas Laughren, M.D., team leader for psychiatric drug products in FDA's division of neuropharmacological drug products.

In the past thirteen years, the Food and Drug Administration has approved several new antidepressants, including Wellbutrin (bupropion), Prozac (fluoxetine), Zoloft (sertraline), Paxil (paroxetine), Effexor (venlafaxine), Serzone (nefazodone), and Remeron (mirtazapine).

According to the American Psychiatric Association (APA), 80 to 90 percent of all cases can be treated effectively. However, two-thirds of the people suffering from depression don't get the help they need, according to NIMH. Many fail to identify their symptoms or attribute them to lack of sleep or a poor diet, the APA says, while others are just too fatigued or ashamed to seek help.

Left untreated, depression can result in years of needless pain for both the depressed person and his or her family. And depression costs the United States an estimated $43 billion a year, due in large part to absenteeism from work, lost productivity, and medical costs, according to the National Depressive and Manic Depressive Association.

Three Types

The three main categories of depression are major depression, dysthymia, and bipolar depression (sometimes referred to as manic depression).

Major depression affects 15 percent of Americans at one point during their lives, according to the U.S. Department of Health and Human Services. Its effects can be so intense that things like eating, sleeping, or just getting out of bed become almost impossible.

Major depression "tends to be a chronic, recurring illness," Laughren explains. Although an individual episode may be treatable, "the majority of people who meet criteria for major depression end up having additional episodes in their lifetime."

Unlike major depression, dysthymia doesn't strike in episodes, but is instead characterized by milder, persistent symptoms that may last for years. Although it usually doesn't interfere with everyday tasks, victims rarely feel like they are functioning at their full capacity. According to the National Alliance for the Mentally Ill, almost 10 million Americans may experience dysthymia each year.

Finally, bipolar disorder cycles between episodes of major depression and highs known as mania. Bipolar disorder is much less common than the other types, afflicting about 1 percent of the U.S. population. Symptoms of mania include irritability, an abnormally elevated mood with a decreased need for sleep, an exaggerated belief in one's own ability, excessive talking, and impulsive and often dangerous behavior.

Genes And Environment

Study after study suggests biochemical and genetic links to depression. A considerable amount of evidence supports the view that depressed people have imbalances in the brain's neurotransmitters, the chemicals that allow communication between nerve cells. Serotonin and norepinephrine are two neurotransmitters whose low levels are thought to play an especially important role. The fact that women have naturally lower serotonin levels than men may contribute to women's greater tendency to depression.

Family histories show a recurrence of depression from generation to generation. Studies of identical twins confirm that depression and genes are related, finding that if one twin of an identical pair suffers from depression, the other has a 70 percent chance of developing the disease. For fraternal twins or siblings, the rate is just 25 percent.

Environmental factors, however, may also play a role in depression. When combined with a biochemical or genetic predisposition, life stressors (such as relationship problems, financial difficulties, death of a loved one, or medical illness) may cause the disease to manifest itself.

John (not his real name), 25, was diagnosed with depression for the first time last year when he and his girlfriend ended their three-year relationship. "I couldn't do anything because I was totally absorbed with the whole break-up issue," he says. "It was impossible for me to sleep, and I would wake up at 3 or 4 in the morning and literally shake. And when it was time to wake up, I just couldn't get out of bed."

In addition, substance abuse and side effects from prescription medication may also lead to a depressive episode. And research shows that people battling serious medical conditions are especially prone to depression. According to the U.S. Department of Health and Human Services, those who have had a heart attack, for example, have a 40 percent chance of being depressed.

Seasonal affective disorder, often called "SAD," is a striking example of an environmental factor playing a major role in depression. SAD usually starts in late fall, with the decrease in daylight hours and ends in spring when the days get longer.

The symptoms of SAD, which include energy loss, increased anxiety, oversleeping, and overeating, may result from a change in the balance of brain chemicals associated with decreased sunlight. The exact reason for the association between light and mood is unknown, but research suggests a connection with the sleep cycle. Several studies have suggested that light therapy, which involves daily exposure to bright fluorescent light, may be an effective treatment for SAD.

Diagnosing The Disease

Medical professionals generally base a diagnosis of depressive disorder on the presence of certain symptoms listed in the American Psychiatric Association's *Diagnostic and Statistical Manual*. The *DSM* lists the following symptoms for depression:

- depressed mood
- loss of interest or pleasure in almost all activities
- changes in appetite or weight
- disturbed sleep
- slowed or restless movements
- fatigue, loss of energy
- feelings of worthlessness or excessive guilt
- trouble in thinking, concentrating, or making decisions
- recurrent thoughts of death or suicide

The diagnosis depends on the number, severity, and duration of these symptoms.

Even with this list of symptoms, diagnosing depression is not simple. According to the National Alliance for the Mentally Ill, it takes an average of eight years from the onset of depression to get a proper diagnosis.

In making a diagnosis, a health professional should also consider the patient's medical history, the findings of a complete physical exam, and laboratory tests to rule out the possibility of depressive symptoms resulting from another medical problem.

The symptoms of the depressive part of bipolar disorder are the same as those expressed in major (unipolar) depression. Because of the similarities in symptoms and the fact that manic episodes usually don't appear until the mid-20s, some people with bipolar disorder may mistakenly be diagnosed with unipolar depression. This may lead to improper treatment because antidepressants carry the risk of triggering a manic episode.

Antidepressant Drugs

One major approach for treating depression is the use of antidepressant medications. The older antidepressants include tricyclic antidepressants such as Tofranil (imipramine) and monoamine oxidase inhibitors such as Nardil (phenelzine). Antidepressants approved more recently include the selective serotonin reuptake inhibitors Prozac, Paxil and Zoloft, and the other newer antidepressants Wellbutrin, Effexor, Serzone, and Remeron.

The effects of antidepressants on the brain are not fully understood, but there is substantial evidence that they somehow restore the brain's chemical balance. These medications usually can control depressive symptoms in four to eight weeks, but many patients remain on antidepressants for six months to a year following a major depressive episode to avoid relapse.

Different drugs work for different people, and it is difficult to predict which people will respond to which drug or who will experience side effects. So it may take more than one try to find the appropriate medication.

Since the mid-1950s, tricyclic antidepressants have been the standard against which other antidepressants have been measured. Monoamine oxidase inhibitors were discovered around the same time as tricyclic antidepressants, but were prescribed less because, if mixed with certain foods or medications, the drugs sometimes resulted in a fatal rise in blood pressure.

Laughren describes Prozac as the "first of a new type of more selective antidepressants." The older antidepressants had unpleasant and sometimes dangerous side effects, such as insomnia, weight gain, blurred vision, sexual impairment, heart palpitations, dry mouth, and constipation. Prozac, other selective serotonin reuptake inhibitors, and other recently approved antidepressants have had generally safer side effect profiles.

A recent study funded by NIMH suggested that Prozac may be as effective in treating children and teens as adults, but the drug is not yet approved by FDA for use in this population.

Other types of therapy, such as natural substances extracted from plants, are currently being studied. Although not approved by FDA, some people believe St. John's wort, for example, is extremely helpful in alleviating their depressive symptoms.

When people are unresponsive to antidepressant medications or can't take them because of their age or health problems, electroconvulsive therapy

✤ **It's A Fact!!**

An Herbal Alternative?

St. John the Baptist's birthday is celebrated on June 24. It is also around this time that the pretty yellow flowers of St. John's wort, the plant named in his honor, bloom in Germany. The plant may be more than just beautiful. Hypericum, the concentrated extract of flowers and leaves, is thought by some to be effective in treating depression.

While the herb is the most-prescribed antidepressant in Germany, in the United States, St. John's wort is not an approved drug. Many health food stores in this country sell it as a dietary supplement, but FDA does not allow any antidepressant claims because it has not been proven to be a safe and effective drug for this use. "There's no particular reason to doubt that it might have biological effects," says Thomas Laughren, M.D., in FDA's division of neuropharmacological drug products. "Whether or not it is an effective antidepressant remains to be seen."

The National Institutes of Health is sponsoring studies to determine if St. John's wort is safe and effective as a treatment for mild to moderate cases of depression. One issue of concern is how the herb interacts with certain drugs, especially antidepressants that affect the brain chemical serotonin.

(ECT), or "shock therapy," can offer a lifesaving alternative. Like anti-depressants, ECT is believed to affect the chemical balance of the brain's neurotransmitters.

Before ECT, the patient is given anesthesia and a muscle relaxant to prevent injury or pain. Then electrodes are placed on the person's head, and a small amount of electricity is applied. This procedure is usually done three times a week until the patient improves. Some patients may experience a temporary loss of short-term memory.

Talking It Out

For severe depressive episodes, medications are often the first step because of the relatively quick relief they can bring to physical symptoms. For the long term, however, psychotherapy may be needed to address certain aspects of the illness that drugs cannot. "Although the biological features of depression may respond better to drugs," Laughren says, "people may need to relearn how to interact with their environment after the biological part of the depression is controlled."

"I wanted to talk things out and get better in that way," John says. "And even after the first couple of times I saw my therapist, I could do a little bit more. Talking with her gave me some reality that how I was feeling wasn't so abnormal, so unusual, or so terrible."

Anne explains, "It's just comforting sometimes to share the little day-to-day happenings in my life with someone who doesn't get to see them first-hand."

Some find support groups to be invaluable in helping them cope with their depression. "It's through talking with others with similar experiences," says Mary Rappaport, "that you can better understand what you're going through."

Changes in lifestyle are also important in the management of depression. Exercise, even in moderate doses, seems to enhance energy and reduce tension. Some research suggests that a rush of the hormone norepinephrine following exercise helps the brain deal with stress that often leads to depression and anxiety. A similar effect may be obtained through meditation, yoga, and certain diets.

A Bright Future

Like many others who have not had to face depression themselves, John's friends lacked knowledge about the disease. "I think the whole thing really affected my relationships with people," he says. "I was pretty much a jerk all of the time. I didn't want to talk to anybody. I just wanted them to leave me alone."

With the growing awareness of the seriousness of the disorder and the biological causes, the understanding and support of family and friends may be easier to come by. "The future looks very bright for individuals who in the past have often had to suffer alone," says Rappaport. "More and more people are coming out, which encourages people to talk about it." Among those who have "come out" recently to publicly discuss their personal bouts with depression are comedian Drew Carey and "60 Minutes" correspondent Mike Wallace.

Experts say that no one, young or old, has to accept feelings of depression as a necessary part of life. The National Depressive and Manic Depressive Association and other organizations offer medical information and referrals. By trying different options for facing their personal challenges, Anne and others have learned what treatments help them most. "All in all," Anne says, "I think my ability to weather the ups and downs of life has gotten better."

Researchers continue to make great strides in understanding and treating depression. For example, scientists are beginning to learn more about the chromosomes where affective disorder genes appear to be located. "While there is a long way to go in coming up with even more effective drugs," Laughren says, "there's much ongoing research and reason for optimism."

If Someone You Know Is Depressed

According to the National Institute of Mental Health, to help someone recover from depression:

- Encourage the person to make an appointment with a doctor, or make the appointment yourself. You may want to go along for support.

- Encourage the person to stick with the treatment plan, including taking prescribed medicine. Improvement may take several weeks. If no improvement occurs, encourage the person to seek a different treatment rather than giving up.

- Give emotional support by listening carefully and offering hope.

- Invite the person to join you in activities that you know he or she used to enjoy, but keep in mind that expecting too much too soon can lead to feelings of failure.

- Do not accuse the person of faking illness or expect them to "snap out of it."

- Take comments about suicide seriously, and seek professional advice.

Where To Go For Help

National Alliance for the Mentally Ill
2107 Wilson Blvd., Suite 300
Arlington, VA 22201
Toll-Free: 800-950-6264
Fax: 703-524-9094
Website: http://www.nami.org

National Depressive and Manic Depressive Association
730 N. Franklin St., Suite 501
Chicago, IL 60610
Toll Free: 800-826-3632
Phone: 312-642-0049
Fax: 312-642-7243
Website: http://www.ndmda.org

National Institute of Mental Health
6001 Executive Boulevard
Rm. 8184, MSC 9663
Rockville, MD 20892-9663
Toll-free 800-64-PANIC (647-2642)
Website: http://www.nimh.nih.gov

☞ **Remember!!**

Depression strikes about 17 million American adults each year, and 80 to 90 percent of all cases can be treated effectively according to the American Psychiatric Association (APA). Yet, two-thirds of the people suffering from depression don't get the help they need. Left untreated, depression can result in years of needless pain for both the depressed person and his or her family.

Chapter 18

Seasonal Affective Disorder

Question

Every winter, especially when the days are short, I feel tired, depressed, and unproductive. Then the spring comes and I start feeling myself again. Is this just a normal seasonal cycle? I've heard about SAD, Seasonal Affective Disorder, but don't know much about it.

Answer

Nobody knows how common Seasonal Affective Disorder (SAD) is, but researchers estimate that it may affect as many as 5 percent of all Americans, or about 14 million people. And many more experience some of these same symptoms, though more or less mildly or consistently—sometimes merely because they work in dark or windowless offices. It's amazing, but it's long been known that the short dark days of winter can cause people to experience a distinctive type of depression and malaise. SAD, in particular, has been defined as follows: fall and winter depressions for at least two years, alternating with non-depressed periods during spring and summer; at least one disabling depressive episode; no other major psychiatric disorder; and no other possible explanation for the mood change.

About This Chapter: Text in this chapter is from "Go Ask Alice!: Seasonal Affective Disorder (SAD)," last updated July 23, 1998, © 1998 by The Trustees of Columbia University in the City of New York. Reprinted with permission.

People with SAD tend to sleep more, be less productive at work, have less energy for recreational activities, including sex, and feel down in the dumps for no particular reason. They tend to eat more (especially sweets and starches) which, together with a low activity level, generally lead to winter weight gain. Generally, the SAD months are November through March, January and February being the worst. Of course, this reflects the population average. At the extremes, annual SAD relapses can begin as early as August and end in January, or they can begin as late as January and last through June. Do not rule SAD out as a possible explanation for the above symptoms if you experience them beginning in, say, October.

✎ Weird Words

Affective Disorder: A mood disorder (pertaining to emotion and feeling) that is not caused by another diagnosable mental disorder.

Seasonal Affective Disorder: A mood disorder that occurs at the same time of the year and gets better as the season changes; common symptoms include depression, fatigue, and a diminished ability to concentrate. Seasonal affective disorder typically occurs during the winter months and symptoms subside in the spring.

If you think you might have SAD, or a milder form of seasonal depression, here are some initial steps you can take, according to the National Institutes of Mental Health (NIMH):

- Make your house, apartment, or room bright. Keep the curtains open. Use bright colors on walls, upholstery, and bedding.

- If you are in an office, ask if you can work near a window.

- Try to go away on vacation in the winter—somewhere sunny and warm!

- Exercise outdoors. If you exercise indoors, try to do so near a window.

Light therapy is another method of SAD treatment. It requires regulated exposure to intense light: a light box consisting of fluorescent bulbs and a diffusion screen. The box is placed on a desk or tabletop where users face the light for about fifteen minutes or more, usually while reading, writing, eating, etc. It is not necessary, or even recommended, to look directly into the light, but the eyes must be open for light therapy to be effective. The degree of light intensity, length of therapy sessions, and the time of day that this treatment is used have a major impact on the success of this treatment, according to preliminary research findings.

For More Information

The resources listed here can provide additional information about light therapy and SAD:

The Center for Environmental Therapeutics (CET)
767 Broadway
Norwood, NJ 07648
Phone: 212-214-0419
Website: http://www.cet.org

Columbia University
308 Low Memorial Library
New York, NY 10027
Phone: 212-854-5017
Clinical Chronogiology Group on line at:
Website: http://www.lightandions.org

The Society for Light Treatment and Biological Rhythms (SLTBR)
842 Howard Avenue
New Haven, CT 06519
Phone: 203-764-4326
Fax: 203-764-4324
Website: http://www.sltbr.org

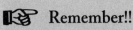 **Remember!!**

If you find that you are unable to remedy your winter depression on your own, you might consider consulting a psychologist or psychiatrist. S/he can coordinate your anti-SAD efforts, from stress management techniques to antidepressants to light therapy.

Chapter 19

Bipolar Disorder

What Is Bipolar Disorder?

Bipolar disorder (also referred to as manic-depressive illness) usually starts in adult life, before the age of 35. Although rare in young children, it can appear both in children and teenagers. This illness can affect anyone. If one or both parents have bipolar disorder, the chances are greater that their children will develop the disorder.

Recognizing The Warning Signs Of Bipolar Disorder

Bipolar disorder may begin with manic or depressive symptoms. The manic symptoms include:

- Severe changes in mood, when compared to peers, either unusually happy or silly, or highly irritable.
- Unrealistic highs in self-esteem.
- Great energy increase; can go with little or no sleep for days without tiring.
- Increased talking—talks too much, too fast; changes topics too quickly; cannot be interrupted.

About This Chapter: The text in this chapter is from "Children's Mental Health: Bipolar Disorder," produced by the National Mental Health Association with support from the William H. Donner Foundation and Eli Lilly and Company, © 1996 National Mental Health Association. Reprinted with permission from the National Mental Health Association (1-800-969-NHMA).

- Distractibility—attention moves constantly from one thing to the next.

- High risk behavior—such as, jumping off a roof and believing no harm will occur to them.

The depressive symptoms include:

- Persistent sadness; frequent crying; depression.

- Loss of enjoyment in favorite activities.

- Frequent physical illnesses—such as, headaches or stomach aches.

- Low energy level—poor concentration, complaining of boredom.

- Major change in eating or sleeping—such as oversleeping or overeating.

✎ Weird Words

Bipolar Disorder: A mood disorder characterized by having cyclical episodes of two extremes—mania (euphoria) and depression; also called manic-depressive disorder.

Depression: A mental condition of emotional dejection, sadness, loneliness, despair, low self-esteem, loss of interest, lack of energy, and withdrawal. Depression can be temporary or chronic.

Irritability: An exaggerated reaction to a stimulus or a quick reaction to annoyance.

Mania: An emotional disorder characterized by a state of excitement, hyperactivity, euphoria, diminished need for sleep, rapid speech, and quickly changing ideas.

Psychotherapy: The treatment of behavioral, emotional, personality, and psychiatric disorders using a variety of psychological methods involving communication between a trained therapist and a person, couple, family, or other group. Forms of psychotherapy include suggestion, hypnotism, and psychoanalysis.

Both bipolar disorder with ADHD (attentive deficit-hyperactivity disorder) and childhood onset bipolar disorder begin early in life and occur mainly in families with a high genetic propensity for both disorders. Adult bipolar disorder is common in both sexes, however most children with bipolar disorder and/or ADHD, are boys.

Children with mania are seldom elated or euphoric; more often they are irritable and subject to outbursts of destructive rage. Childhood bipolar symptoms are often chronic and continuous rather than acute and episodic, as in adults. Bipolar disorder may account for a large proportion of children's psychiatric hospitalizations.

♣ **It's A Fact!!**

Diagnosis of bipolar disorder in teens can be complicated because its symptoms can also be symptoms of depression, conduct disorder, stress responses, drug abuse, delinquency, attention-deficit hyperactivity disorder, or schizophrenia.

Teens also have an ongoing combination of extremely high (manic) and low (depressive) moods. Highs may alternate with lows, or the person may feel both extremes almost simultaneously.

Confusion With Other Problems

Irritability and aggressiveness in children complicate the diagnosis, since they can also be symptoms of depression or conduct disorder, or even normal responses to stress. The irritability of bipolar children is especially severe and often leads to violence. The aggressiveness may suggest a conduct disorder, although it is usually less organized and purposeful than the aggression of predatory juvenile delinquents.

These signs are also similar to common teen problems such as, drug abuse, delinquency, attention-deficit hyperactivity disorder, or even schizophrenia. The diagnosis requires careful observation over an extended time period. An evaluation by a child and adolescent psychiatrist can be helpful in identifying the problem, whether it is bipolar disorder or other mental health illness;

and for starting specific treatment. Some children with bipolar disorder (or a combination of bipolar and ADHD) may be diagnosed as having only ADHD. The two disorders appear to be genetically linked.

Treatment Of The Bipolar Disorder

In children, unstable moods—which are generally the most serious problem—should be treated first. Not much can be done about ADHD while the child is subject to extreme mood swings.

Teens with bipolar disorder can be effectively treated. Treatment usually includes:

- psychotherapy which helps the teen adapt to stress; to rebuild self-esteem and to improve relationships.
- medications which often reduce the frequency and severity of manic episodes and help to prevent depression.
- education of the entire family about the illness.

For More Information

For more information about bipolar disorder, contact your local Mental Health Association, community mental health center, or:

National Mental Health Association
1021 Prince St.
Alexandria, VA 22314-2971
Toll-Free: 800-969-6642
Website: http://www.nmha.org

American Association of Suicidology
4201 Connecticut Avenue, N.W.
Suite 408
Washington, DC 20008
Phone: 202-237-2280
Fax: 202-237-2282
Website: http://www.suicidology.org

American Academy of Child and Adolescent Psychiatry
3615 Wisconsin Avenue, N.W.
Washington, DC 20016
Phone: 202-966-7300
Fax: 202-966-2891
Website: http://www.aacap.org

☞ **Remember!!**

Although bipolar disorder is generally
found in adults, it can occur in teens. Effective treatment includes both medications and therapy.

Chapter 20

Early-Onset Bipolar Disorder

Bipolar disorder (also known as manic-depression) is a serious but treatable medical illness. It is a disorder of the brain marked by extreme changes in mood, energy, and behavior. Symptoms may be present since infancy or early childhood, or may suddenly emerge in adolescence or adulthood. Until recently, a diagnosis of the disorder was rarely made in childhood. Doctors can now recognize and treat bipolar disorder in young children.

Early intervention and treatment offer the best chance for children with emerging bipolar disorder to achieve stability, gain the best possible level of wellness, and grow up to enjoy their gifts and build upon their strengths. Proper treatment can minimize the adverse effects of the illness on their lives and the lives of those who love them.

Families of affected children and adolescents are almost always baffled by early-onset bipolar disorder and are desperate for information and support.

About This Chapter: Text in this chapter is from "About Early-Onset Bipolar Disorder," by the Child and Adolescent Bipolar Foundation (CABF) posted at http://www.bpkids.org/learning/about.htm. The article was reviewed by Demitri Papolos, M.D., Chairman, CABF Professional Advisory Board and edited by Martha Hellander, CABF Executive Director. © CABF 2000; reprinted with permission.

Common Questions Asked About The Disorder

How Common Is Bipolar Disorder In Children?

It is not known, because studies are lacking. However, bipolar disorder affects an estimated 1-2 percent of adults worldwide. The more we learn about this disorder, the more prevalent it appears to be among children.

• It is suspected that a significant number of children diagnosed in the United States with attention-deficit disorder with hyperactivity (ADHD) have early-onset bipolar disorder instead of, or along with, ADHD.

✎ Weird Words

Attention-Deficit Hyperactivity Disorder (ADHD): A behavioral disorder characterized by a pattern of inattention, excessive activity, learning disabilities, and disruptive behavior which is usually observed in family, school, and social settings.

Depression: A mental condition of emotional dejection, sadness, loneliness, despair, low self-esteem, loss of interest, lack of energy, and withdrawal. Depression can be temporary or chronic.

Diagnostic and Statistical Manual IV (DSM-IV): Complete title of this book, which is produced by the American Psychiatric Association, is Diagnostic and Statistical Manual of Mental Disorders, Fourth Edition. It provides standard names and descriptions of mental disorders; these terms and guidelines are used by health care providers in making diagnostic assessments. The first edition was published in 1952; the fourth edition, which is the most recent, was published in 1994.

Lithium: A medication used in the treatment of mental illness, especially the manic phases of bipolar disorder.

Mania: An emotional disorder characterized by a state of excitement, hyperactivity, euphoria, diminished need for sleep, rapid speech, and quickly changing ideas.

- According to the American Academy of Child and Adolescent Psychiatry, up to one-third of the 3.4 million children and adolescents with depression in the United States may actually be experiencing the early onset of bipolar disorder.

What Are The Symptoms Of Bipolar Disorder In Children?

Bipolar disorder involves marked changes in mood and energy. In most adults with the illness, persistent states of extreme elation or agitation accompanied by high energy are called mania. Persistent states of extreme sadness or irritability accompanied by low energy are called depression.

However, the illness looks different in children than it does in adults. Children usually have an ongoing, continuous mood disturbance that is a mix of mania and depression. This rapid and severe cycling between moods produces chronic irritability and few clear periods of wellness between episodes.

Symptoms of bipolar disorder can emerge as early as infancy. Mothers often report that children later diagnosed with the disorder were extremely difficult to settle and slept erratically. They seemed extraordinarily clingy, and from a very young age often had uncontrollable, seizure-like tantrums or rages out of proportion to any event. The word "no" often triggered these rages.

Several ongoing studies are further exploring characteristics of affected children. Researchers are studying, with promising results, the effectiveness and safety of adult treatments in children.

What Are The Symptoms Of Bipolar Disorder In Adolescents?

In adolescents, bipolar disorder may resemble any of the following classical adult presentations of the illness.

- **Bipolar I.** In this form of the disorder, the adolescent experiences alternating episodes of intense and sometimes psychotic mania and depression. Periods of relative or complete wellness occur between the episodes.

Symptoms of mania include:

- elevated, expansive or irritable mood
- decreased need for sleep
- racing speech and pressure to keep talking
- grandiose delusions
- excessive involvement in pleasurable but risky activities
- increased physical and mental activity
- poor judgment
- in severe cases, hallucinations

Symptoms of depression include:

- pervasive sadness and crying spells
- sleeping too much or inability to sleep
- agitation and irritability
- withdrawal from activities formerly enjoyed
- drop in grades and inability to concentrate
- thoughts of death and suicide
- low energy
- significant change in appetite

- **Bipolar II.** In this form of the disorder, the adolescent experiences episodes of hypomania between recurrent periods of depression. Hypomania is a markedly elevated or irritable mood accompanied by increased physical and mental energy. Hypomania can be a time of great creativity.

- **Cyclothymia.** Adolescents with this form of the disorder experience periods of less severe, but definite, mood swings.

- **Bipolar Disorder NOS (Not Otherwise Specified).** Doctors make this diagnosis when it is not clear which type of bipolar disorder is emerging.

For some adolescents, a loss or other traumatic event may trigger a first episode of depression or mania. Later episodes may occur independently of any obvious stresses, or may worsen with stress. Puberty is a time of risk. In girls, the onset of menses may trigger the illness, and symptoms often vary in severity with the monthly cycle.

Once the illness starts, episodes tend to recur and worsen without treatment. Studies show that after symptoms first appear, typically there is a 10-year lag until treatment begins. Child and Adolescent Bipolar Foundation (CABF) encourages parents to take their adolescent for an evaluation if four or more of the above symptoms persist for more than two weeks. Early intervention and treatment can make all the difference in the world during this critical time of development.

Are Substance Abuse And Addiction Related To Bipolar Disorder?

A majority of teens with untreated bipolar disorder abuse alcohol and drugs. Any child or adolescent who abuses substances should be evaluated for a mood disorder.

Adolescents who seemed normal until puberty and experience a comparatively sudden onset of symptoms are thought to be especially vulnerable to developing addiction to drugs or alcohol. Substances may be readily available among their peers and teens may use them to attempt to control their mood swings and insomnia. If addiction develops, it is essential to treat both the bipolar disorder and the substance abuse at the same time.

What Role Does Genetics Or Family History Play In Bipolar Disorder?

The illness tends to be highly genetic, but there are clearly environmental factors that influence whether the illness will occur in a particular child. Bipolar disorder can skip generations and take different forms in different individuals.

The small group of studies that have been done vary in the estimate of risk to a given individual:

• For the general population, a conservative estimate of an individual's risk of having full-blown bipolar disorder is 1 percent. Disorders in the bipolar spectrum may affect 4-6%.

- When one parent has bipolar disorder, the risk to each child is 15-30%.

- When both parents have bipolar disorder, the risk increases to 50-75%.

- The risk in siblings and fraternal twins is 15-25%.

- The risk in identical twins is approximately 70%.

In every generation since World War II, there is a higher incidence and an earlier age of onset of bipolar disorder and depression. On average, children with bipolar disorder experience their first episode of illness 10 years earlier than their parents' generation did. The reason for this is unknown.

The family trees of many children who develop early-onset bipolar disorder include individuals who suffered from substance abuse and/or mood disorders (often undiagnosed). Also among their relatives are found highly-accomplished, creative, and extremely successful individuals in business, politics, and the arts.

✔ **Quick Tip**

Symptoms of bipolar disorder may include:

- an expansive or irritable mood

- depression

- rapidly changing moods lasting a few hours to a few days

- explosive, lengthy, and often destructive rages

- separation anxiety

- defiance of authority

- hyperactivity, agitation, and distractibility

- sleeping little or, alternatively, sleeping too much

- bed wetting and night terrors

- strong and frequent cravings, often for carbohydrates and sweets

- excessive involvement in multiple projects and activities

- impaired judgment, impulsivity, racing thoughts, and pressure to keep talking

- dare-devil behaviors

- inappropriate or precocious sexual behavior

- delusions and hallucinations

- grandiose belief in own abilities that defy the laws of logic (ability to fly, for example)

Diagnosing Bipolar Disorder In Children

Healthy children often have moments when they have difficulty staying still, controlling their impulses, or dealing with frustration. The *Diagnostic and Statistical Manual IV* (*DSM-IV*) still requires that, for a diagnosis of bipolar disorder, adult criteria must be met. There are as yet no separate criteria for diagnosing children.

Some behaviors by a child, however, should raise a red flag:

• destructive rages that continue past the age of four

• talk of wanting to die or kill themselves

• trying to jump out of a moving car

To illustrate how difficult it is to use the *DSM-IV* to diagnose children, the manual says that a hypomanic episode requires a "distinct period of persistently elevated, expansive, or irritable mood lasting throughout at least four days." Yet upwards of 70 percent of children with the illness have mood and energy shifts several times a day.

Since the *DSM-IV* is not scheduled for revision in the immediate future, experts often use some *DSM-IV* criteria as well as other measures. For example, a Washington University team of researchers uses a structured diagnostic interview called Wash U KIDDE-SADS, which is more sensitive to the rapid-cycling periods commonly observed in children with bipolar disorder.

How Does Bipolar Disorder Differ From Other Conditions?

Even when a child's behavior is unquestionably not normal, correct diagnosis remains challenging. Bipolar disorder is often accompanied by symptoms of other psychiatric disorders. In some children, proper treatment for the bipolar disorder clears up the troublesome symptoms thought to indicate another diagnosis. In other children, bipolar disorder may explain only part of a more complicated case that includes neurological, developmental, and other components.

Diagnoses that mask or sometimes occur along with bipolar disorder include:

- depression
- conduct disorder (CD)
- oppositional-defiant disorder (ODD)
- attention-deficit disorder with hyperactivity (ADHD)
- panic disorder
- generalized anxiety disorder (GAD)
- obsessive-compulsive disorder (OCD)
- Tourette's syndrome (TS)
- intermittent explosive disorder
- reactive attachment disorder (RAD)

In adolescents, bipolar disorder is often misdiagnosed as:

- borderline personality disorder
- post-traumatic stress disorder (PTSD)
- schizophrenia

The Need For Prompt And Proper Diagnosis

Tragically, after symptoms first appear in children, years often pass before treatment begins, if ever. Meanwhile, the disorder worsens and the child's functioning at home, school, and in the community is progressively more impaired.

The importance of proper diagnosis cannot be overstated. The results of untreated or improperly treated bipolar disorder can include:

- an unnecessary increase in symptomatic behaviors leading to removal from school, placement in a residential treatment center, hospitalization in a psychiatric hospital, or incarceration in the juvenile justice system
- the development of personality disorders such as narcissistic, antisocial, and borderline personality
- a worsening of the disorder due to incorrect medications
- drug abuse, accidents, and suicide.

It is important to remember that a diagnosis is not a scientific fact. It is a considered opinion based upon the behavior of the child over time, what is known of the child's family history, the child's response to medications, his or her developmental stage, the current state of scientific knowledge and the training and experience of the doctor making the diagnosis. These factors (and the diagnosis) can change as more information becomes available. Competent professionals can disagree on which diagnosis fits an individual best. Diagnosis is important, however, because it guides treatment decisions and allows the family to put a name to the condition that affects their child. Diagnosis can provide answers to some questions but raises others that are unanswerable given the current state of scientific knowledge.

How Can Parents Help A Child?

Parents concerned about their child's behavior, especially suicidal talk and gestures, should have the child immediately evaluated by a professional familiar with the symptoms and treatment of early-onset bipolar disorder.

There is no a blood test or brain scan, as yet, that can establish a diagnosis of bipolar disorder.

✤ It's A Fact!!

Bipolar disorder has left its mark on history. Many famous and accomplished people had symptoms of the illness, including:

- Abraham Lincoln
- Winston Churchill
- Theodore Roosevelt
- Goethe
- Balzac
- Handel
- Schumann
- Berlioz
- Tolstoy
- Virginia Woolf
- Hemingway
- Robert Lowell
- Anne Sexton

The biographies of Beethoven, Newton, and Dickens, in particular, reveal severe and debilitating recurrent mood swings beginning in childhood.

Parents who suspect that their child has bipolar disorder (or any psychiatric illness) should take daily notes of their child's mood, behavior, sleep patterns, unusual events, and statements by the child of concern to the parents. Share these notes with the doctor making the evaluation and with the doctor who eventually treats your child. Some parents fax or e-mail a copy of their notes to the doctor before each appointment.

Because children with bipolar disorder can be charming and charismatic during an appointment, they initially may appear to a professional to be functioning well. Therefore, a good evaluation takes at least two appointments and includes a detailed family history.

Finding The Right Doctor

If possible, look for a board-certified child psychiatrist. A child psychiatrist is a medical doctor who has completed two to three years of an adult psychiatric residency and two additional years of a child psychiatry fellowship program. Unfortunately, there is a severe shortage of child psychiatrists, and few have extensive experience treating early-onset bipolar disorder.

Teaching hospitals affiliated with reputable medical schools are often a good place to start looking for an experienced child psychiatrist. You can also ask your pediatrician for a referral. The American Academy of Child and Adolescent Psychiatry has a searchable database of their members. Some doctors list a special interest in bipolar disorder.

If your community does not have a child psychiatrist with expertise in mood disorders, then look for an adult psychiatrist who has 1) a broad background in mood disorders, and 2) experience in treating children and adolescents.

Other specialists who may be able to help, at least with an initial evaluation, include pediatric neurologists. Neurologists have experience with the anti-convulsant medications often used for treating juvenile bipolar disorders. Pediatricians who consult with a psychopharmacologist can also provide competent care if a child psychiatrist is not available.

Some families take their child to nationally-known doctors at teaching hospitals for diagnosis and stabilization. They then turn to local professionals for medical management of their child's treatment and psychotherapy. The local professionals consult with the expert as needed.

Treatment

Although there is no cure for bipolar disorder, in most cases treatment can stabilize mood and allow for management and control of symptoms.

A good treatment plan includes medication, close monitoring of symptoms, education about the illness, counseling or psychotherapy for the individual and family, stress reduction, good nutrition, regular sleep and exercise, and participation in a network of support.

✔ **Quick Tip**

Experienced parents recommend that you look for a doctor who:

- is knowledgeable about mood disorders, has a strong background in psychopharmacology, and stays up-to-date on the latest research in the field

- knows he or she does not have all the answers and welcomes information discovered by the parents

- explains medical matters clearly, listens well, and returns phone calls promptly

- offers to work closely with parents and values their input

- has a good rapport with the child

- understands how traumatic a hospitalization is for both child and parents, and keeps in touch with the family during this period

- advocates for the child with managed care companies when necessary

- advocates for the child with the school to make sure the child receives services appropriate to the child's educational needs.

The good news is that with appropriate treatment and support at home and at school, many children with bipolar disorder achieve a marked reduction in the severity, frequency and duration of episodes of illness. With education about their illness (as is provided to children with epilepsy, diabetes, and other chronic conditions) they learn how to manage and monitor their symptoms as they grow older.

The Parent's Role In Treatment

As with other chronic medical conditions such as diabetes, epilepsy, and asthma, children and adolescents with bipolar disorder and their families need to work closely with their doctor and other treatment professionals. Having the entire family involved in the child's treatment plan can usually reduce the frequency, duration, and severity of episodes. It can also help improve the child's ability to function successfully at home, in school, and in the community.

♣ It's A Fact!!

In treating bipolar disorder in children and adolescents, the response to medications and treatment varies. Factors that contribute to a better outcome are:

- access to competent medical care
- early diagnosis and treatment
- adherence to medication and treatment plan
- a flexible, low-stress home and school environment
- a supportive network of family and friends

Factors that complicate treatment are:

- lack of access to competent medical care
- time lag between onset of illness and treatment
- not taking prescribed medications
- stressful and inflexible home and school environment
- the co-occurrence of other diagnoses
- use of substances such as illegal drugs and alcohol

Medication

Few controlled studies have been done on the use of psychiatric medications in children. The U.S. Food and Drug Administration (FDA) has approved only a handful for pediatric use. Psychiatrists must adapt what they know about treating adults to children and adolescents.

Medications used to treat adults are often helpful in stabilizing mood in children. Most doctors start medication immediately upon diagnosis if both parents agree. If one parent disagrees, a short period of watchful waiting and charting of symptoms can be helpful. Treatment should not be postponed for long, however, because of the risk of suicide and school failure.

A symptomatic child should never be left unsupervised. If parental disagreement makes treatment impossible, as may happen in families undergoing divorce, a court order regarding treatment may be necessary.

Other treatments, such as psychotherapy, may not be effective until mood stabilization occurs. In fact, stimulants and antidepressants given without a mood stabilizer (often the result of misdiagnosis) can cause havoc in bipolar children, potentially inducing mania, more frequent cycling, and increases in aggressive outbursts.

No one medication works in all children. The family should expect a trial-and-error process lasting weeks, months, or longer as doctors try several medications alone and in combination before they find the best treatment. It is important not to become discouraged during the initial treatment phase. Two or more mood stabilizers, plus additional medications for symptoms that remain, are often necessary to achieve and maintain stability.

Parents often find it hard to accept that their child has a chronic condition that may require treatment with several medications. It is important to remember that untreated bipolar disorder has a fatality rate of 18 percent or more (from suicide), equal to or greater than that for many serious physical illnesses. The untreated disorder carries the risk of drug and alcohol addiction, damaged relationships, school failure, and difficulty finding and holding jobs. The risks of not treating are substantial and must be measured against the unknown risks of using medications whose safety and efficacy have been established in adults, but not yet in children.

The following is a brief overview of medications used to treat bipolar disorder. This brief overview is not intended to replace the evaluation and treatment of any child by a physician. Be sure to consult with a doctor who knows your child before starting, stopping, or changing any medication.

> ✔ Quick Tip
>
> **For Parents:** Learn all you can about bipolar disorder. Read, join support groups, and network with other parents. There are many questions still unanswered about early onset bipolar disorder, but early intervention and treatment can often stabilize mood and restore wellness. You can best manage relapses by prompt intervention at the first re-occurrence of symptoms.

Mood Stabilizers

- Lithium (Eskalith, Lithobid, lithium carbonate)—A salt that occurs naturally in the earth, lithium has been used successfully for decades to calm mania and prevent mood cycling. Lithium has a proven anti-suicidal effect. An estimated 70 to 80 percent of adult bipolar patients respond positively to lithium treatment. Some children do well on lithium, but others do better on other mood stabilizers. Lithium is often used in combination with another mood stabilizer.

- Divalproex sodium or valproic acid (Depakote)—Doctors frequently prescribe this anti-convulsant for children who have rapid cycling between mania and depression.

- Carbamazepine (Tegretol)—Doctors prescribe this anti-convulsant because of its anti-manic and anti-aggressive properties. It is useful in treating frequent rage attacks.

- Gabapentin (Neurontin)—This is a newer anti-convulsant drug that seems to have fewer side effects than other mood stabilizers. However,

doctors do not know how effective this drug is, and some parents report activation of manic symptoms in young children.

- Lamotrigine (Lamictal)—This newer anti-convulsant medicine can
  be effective in controlling rapid cycling. It seems to work well in the
  depressive, as well as the manic, phase of bipolar disorder. Any appearance of rash must be immediately reported to the doctor, as a rare but
  severe side-effect may occur (for this reason Lamictal is not used in
  children under 16).

- Topiramate (Topamax)—This newer anti-convulsant drug may control rapid-cycling and mixed bipolar states in patients who have not
  responded well to divalproex sodium or carbamazepine. Unlike other
  mood stabilizers, it does not have weight gain as a side effect, but its
  efficacy in children has not been established.

- Tiagabine (Gabitrol)—This newer anti-convulsant drug has FDA
  approval for use in adolescents and is now being used in children as
  well.

Other Medications

Doctors may prescribe antipsychotic medications (Risperdal, Zyprexa,
Seroquel) for use during manic states, particularly when children experience
delusions or hallucinations and when rapid control of mania is needed. Some
of the newer antipsychotic medications are very effective in controlling rages
and aggression. Weight gain is often a side effect of anti-psychotic medications.

Calcium channel blockers (verapamil, nimodipine, isradipine) have recently received attention as potential mood stabilizers for treating acute mania,
ultra-ultra-rapid cycling, and recurrent depression.

Anti-anxiety medications (Klonopin, Xanax, Buspar, and Ativan) decrease
anxiety by diminishing activity in brain arousal systems. They reduce agitation and over-activity, and help promote standard sleep. Doctors commonly
use these medications as add-ons to mood stabilizers and antipsychotic drugs
in acute mania.

Alternative And Supplemental Treatments

Alternative and supplemental treatments, such as light therapy, electro-convulsive therapy, transcranial magnetic stimulation, and nutritional supplements, such as Omega-3 oil (fish oil) and St. John's Wort are sometimes used for treating bipolar disorder. (Some reports indicate that St. John's Wort can trigger mania; it should not be administered to children.)

Psychotherapy

In addition to seeing a child psychiatrist, the treatment plan for a child with bipolar disorder usually includes regular therapy sessions with a licensed clinical social worker, a licensed psychologist, or a psychiatrist who provides psychotherapy. Cognitive behavioral therapy, interpersonal therapy, and multi-family support groups are an essential part of treatment for children and adolescents with bipolar disorder. A support group for the child or adolescent with the disorder can also be beneficial, although few exist.

Therapeutic Parenting™

Parents of children with bipolar disorder have discovered numerous techniques that the CABF refers to as therapeutic parenting. These techniques help calm their children when they are symptomatic and can help prevent and contain relapses. Such techniques include:

- practicing and teaching their child relaxation techniques
- using firm restraint holds to contain rages
- prioritizing battles and letting go of less important matters
- reducing stress in the home, including learning and using good listening and communication skills
- using music and sound, lighting, water, and massage to assist the child with waking, falling asleep, and relaxation
- becoming an advocate for stress reduction and other accommodations at school
- helping the child anticipate and avoid, or prepare for stressful situations by developing coping strategies beforehand

- engaging the child's creativity through activities that express and channel their gifts and strengths

- providing routine structure and a great deal of freedom within limits

- removing objects from the home (or locking them in a safe place) that could be used to harm self or others during a rage, especially guns; keeping medications in a locked cabinet or box.

Educational Needs Of A Child With Bipolar Disorder

A diagnosis of bipolar disorder means the child has a significant health impairment (such as diabetes, epilepsy, or leukemia) that requires ongoing medical management. The child needs and is entitled to accommodations in school to benefit from his or her education. Bipolar disorder and the medications used to treat it can affect a child's school attendance, alertness and concentration, sensitivity to light, noise and stress, motivation, and energy available for learning. The child's functioning can vary greatly at different times throughout the day, season, and school year.

The special education staff, parents and professionals should meet as a team to determine the child's educational needs. An evaluation including psychoeducational testing will be done by the school (some families arrange for more extensive private testing). The educational needs of a particular child with bipolar disorder vary depending on the frequency, severity, and duration of episodes of illness. These factors are difficult to predict in an individual case. Transitions to new teachers and new schools, return to school from vacations and absences, and changing to new medications are common times of increased symptoms for children with bipolar disorder. Medication side effects that can be troublesome at school include increased thirst and urination, excessive sleepiness or agitation, and interference with concentration. Weight gain, fatigue, and a tendency to become easily overheated and dehydrated impact a child's participation in gym and regular classes.

These factors and any others that affect the child's education must be identified. A plan (called an IEP) will be written to accommodate the child's needs. The IEP should include accommodations for periods when the child is relatively well (when a less intense level of services may suffice), and accommodations available to the child in the event of relapse. Specific accommodations should be backed up by a letter or phone call from the child's doctor to the director of special education in the school district. Some parents find it necessary to hire a lawyer to obtain the accommodations and services that federal law requires public schools to provide for children with similar health impairments.

Examples of accommodations helpful to children and adolescents with bipolar disorder include:

- preschool special education testing and services

- small class size (with children of similar intelligence) or self-contained classroom with other emotionally fragile (not "behavior disorder") children for part or all of the day

- one-on-one or shared special education aide to assist child in class

- back-and-forth notebook between home and school to assist communication

- homework reduced or excused and deadlines extended when energy is low

- late start to school day if fatigued in morning

- recorded books as alternative to self-reading when concentration is low

☞ Remember!!

Learning that one has bipolar disorder can be traumatic. Diagnosis usually follows months or years of the child's mood instability, school difficulties, and damaged relationships with family and friends. However, diagnosis can and should be a turning point for everyone concerned. Once the illness is identified, energies can be directed towards treatment, education, and developing coping strategies.

For further information, contact:

Child and Adolescent Bipolar Foundation
1187 Wilmett Avenue
PMB #331
Wilmett, IL 60091
Phone: 847-256-8525
Fax: 847-920-9498

Website: www.bpkids.org
E-Mail: cabf@bpkids.org

- designation of a "safe place" at school where child can retreat when overwhelmed

- designation of a staff member to whom the child can go as needed

- unlimited access to bathroom

- unlimited access to drinking water

- art therapy and music therapy

- extended time on tests

- use of calculator for math

- extra set of books at home

- use of keyboard or dictation for writing assignments

- regular sessions with a social worker or school psychologist

- social skills groups and peer support groups

- annual in-service training for teachers by child's treatment professionals (sponsored by school)

- enriched art, music, or other areas of particular strength

- curriculum that engages creativity and reduces boredom (for highly creative children)

- tutoring during extended absences

- goals set each week with rewards for achievement

- summer services such as day camps and special education summer school

- placement in a day hospital treatment program for periods of acute illness that can be managed without inpatient hospitalization

- placement in a therapeutic day school during extended relapses or to provide a period of extra support after hospitalization and before returning to regular school

- placement in a residential treatment center during extended periods of illness if a therapeutic day school near the family's home is not available or is unable to meet the child's needs

Chapter 21

Anxiety Disorders

What Are Anxiety Disorders?

Arousal and stress reactions are essential for human survival; they enable people to pursue important goals and to respond appropriately to danger. In a healthy individual, the stress response (fight, fright, or flight) is provoked by a genuine threat or challenge and is used as a spur for appropriate action. Anxiety, however, is excessive or inappropriate arousal characterized by feelings of apprehension, uncertainty, and fear. The word is derived from the Latin, angere, which means to choke or strangle. It is often not attributable to a real or appropriate threat but it can paralyze the individual into inaction or withdrawal. An anxiety disorder also persists.

Anxiety disorders are the most common psychiatric condition in the United States. About 25 million Americans experience anxiety disorders at some time during their lives; the lifetime risk for an anxiety disorder is nearly 25%. Nevertheless, only about a quarter of those who experience this problem seek help. In recent years, a number of different anxiety disorders have been classified; the two primary ones are generalized anxiety disorder (GAD), which is long-lasting and low-grade, and panic disorder, which has more

About This Chapter: The text in this chapter is from "The Well-Connected Guide to Anxiety," located at www.well-connected.com © 2000 Nidus Information Services, Inc. Reprinted with permission.

dramatic symptoms. Other anxiety disorders include phobias, performance anxiety, obsessive-compulsive disorder (OCD), and post-traumatic stress disorder (PTSD). Anxiety disorders are usually caused by a combination of psychological, physical, and genetic conditions, and treatment is, in general, very effective.

✎ Weird Words

Anxiety: An emotional state characterized by apprehension, uneasiness, dread of impending danger, or fear; often accompanied by symptoms such as a rapid heartbeat, agitation, tension, and restlessness.

Anxiety Disorder: A type of mental disorder involving exaggerated and un-controllable reactions to stress which interfere with normal life functioning. Frequently the source of these feelings is nonspecific or not consciously known by the patient. Panic disorders, simple phobias, social phobia, and obsessive-compulsive disorder are all examples of anxiety disorders.

Arousal: A state of alertness or being prepared to act.

Compulsion: Uncontrollable impulses to perform a certain act for the purpose of alleviating fear or anxiety.

Generalized Anxiety Disorder: A mental disorder characterized by chronic and excessive reactions of anxiety, fear, and dread with symp-toms that can include restlessness, fatigue, and irritability.

Obsessive-Compulsive Disorder: A mental disorder characterized by the persistent intrusion of unwanted ideas and the compulsion to perform repetitive, time-consuming acts (such as handwashing or touching) or ritualistic behaviors to relieve anxiety.

Panic: Sudden, overwhelming fear or anxiety that is extreme and unrea-sonable, often accompanied by symptoms such as an increased heart rate, rapid breathing, and sweating.

What Are The Symptoms Of Anxiety?

Physically, anxiety is usually expressed through a series of responses that include a rise in blood pressure, a fast heart rate, rapid breathing, and an increase in muscle tension; intestinal blood flow decreases, sometimes resulting in nausea or diarrhea. Specific anxiety disorders are diagnosed based

Panic Attack: A period of intense fear or anxiety accompanied by symptoms such as shortness of breath, heart palpitations, sweating, trembling, chest pain, dizziness, and fear of losing control.

Phobia: An abnormal, persistent, irrational fear or dread that causes a state of panic.

Post-Traumatic Stress Disorder: A mental disorder with distinguishing symptoms following a traumatic event. The symptoms of post-traumatic stress disorder include re-experiencing the event, avoiding things associated with the event, dysfunctional thought processes, numbing of general responses, increased arousal, heightened startle reflex, insomnia, and nightmares.

Social Phobia: Fear and resulting avoidance of social situations in which a person would be noticed. One of the most common social phobias is the fear of public speaking.

Tic: An involuntary, brief, and recurrent twitching of a group of muscles, typically involving the face, mouth, eyes, head, neck, or shoulders. Tics are habitual actions that can be deliberately suppressed only for short periods of time

Tourette's Syndrome: A generalized tic disorder, usually beginning in childhood, characterized by facial and vocal tics, continuous gestures, facial twitching, uncontrollable use of foul language, and repetition of things spoken by others.

on the severity and duration of symptoms and on additional behavioral characteristics that accompany the symptoms of anxiety.

Generalized Anxiety Disorder Symptoms

Generalized anxiety disorder (GAD), which affects about 10 million Americans, is characterized by a more-or-less constant state of tension and anxiety over various situations; this state lasts more than six months despite the lack of an obvious or specific stressor. It is very difficult to control worry. (For a clear diagnosis of GAD, these worries are not the same as those of other anxiety disorders, such as fear of panic attacks or appearing in public, nor are they obsessive as in obsessive-compulsive disorder. It should be noted, however, that over half of those with GAD also have another anxiety disorder or depression.) Given these conditions, a diagnosis of GAD is confirmed if three or more of the following symptoms are present (only one for children): feeling on edge or very restless, feeling tired, having difficulty with concentration, feeling irritable, having muscle tension, experiencing sleep disturbances. Some of these symptoms occur on most days for six months. Symptoms should cause significant distress and impair normal functioning and not be due to a medical condition or other mood disorder or psychosis.

❖ **It's A Fact!!**

An estimated 25 million Americans will experience anxiety disorders at some time during their lives. The most common of the anxiety disorders is generalized anxiety disorder, which affects about 10 million Americans.

Panic Disorder Symptoms

Panic disorder is characterized by periodic attacks of anxiety or terror, which usually last 15 to 30 minutes, although residual effects can persist much longer. The frequency and severity of acute states of anxiety determine the diagnosis. During a panic attack a person feels intense fear or discomfort with at least four or more of the following symptoms: rapid heart beat, sweating, shakiness, shortness of breath, a choking feeling, dizziness, nausea, feelings of unreality, numbness, either hot flashes or chills, chest pain, fear of dying, and fear of going insane. A diagnosis of panic disorder is made when a person experiences at least two recurrent, unexpected panic attacks followed by at least one month of fear that another will occur. Frequency of attacks can vary widely. Some people have frequent attacks (for example, every week) that occur for months; others may have clusters of daily attacks followed by weeks or months of remission. Panic attacks may occur spontaneously or in response to a particular situation. If the patient associates fear with harmless circumstances surrounding the original attack, similar circumstances later on may recall the anxiety and trigger additional panic attacks. Panic attacks that include only one or two symptoms, such as dizziness and heart pounding, are known as limited-symptom attacks; these may be either residual symptoms after a major panic attack or precursors to full-blown attacks. (It should be noted that panic attacks occur with other anxiety disorders, including phobias and post-traumatic stress disorder.)

Phobic Disorders Symptoms

Phobias, overwhelming and irrational fears, are common, but they vary in severity. In most cases, people can avoid or at least endure phobic situations, but in some cases, as with agoraphobia, the anxiety associated with the feared object or situation can be incapacitating.

Agoraphobia. About half of people with panic disorders develop agoraphobia, which has been somewhat misleadingly described as fear of open spaces, the term having been derived from the Greek word *agora* meaning marketplace. In its severest form, agoraphobia is characterized by a paralyzing terror of being in places or situations from which the patient feels there is no escape or accessible help in case of an attack. (One patient described the terror of going outside as opening a door onto a landscape filled with snakes.) Consequently, agoraphobes confine themselves to places in which they feel safe, usually at home. The patient with agoraphobia often makes complicated plans in order to avoid confronting feared situations and places.

Social Phobia And Performance Anxiety. Social phobia is the fear of being publicly scrutinized and humiliated and is manifested by extreme shyness and discomfort in social settings. The associated symptoms vary in intensity, ranging from mild and tolerable anxiety to a full-blown panic attack; symptoms include sweating, shortness of breath, pounding heart, dry mouth, and tremor. The disorder is defined as generalized or specific. Generalized social phobia includes fear of being humiliated in front of other people while doing various activities, such as writing in the presence of others or urinating in a public bathroom. Specific social activity usually involves a phobic response to a specific event. For example, performance anxiety, or stage fright, is a specific social phobia that occurs when a person must perform in public. The incidence of social phobia is approximately 13% and has been termed "the neglected anxiety disorder" because it is often missed as a diagnosis.

Simple Phobias. A simple phobia is an irrational fear of specific objects or situations. The most common phobias are fear of animals (usually spiders, snakes, or mice), flying (pterygophobia), heights (acrophobia), water, public transportation, confined spaces (claustrophobia), dentists (odontiatophobia), storms, tunnels, and bridges. When confronting the object or situation, the phobic person experiences panicky feelings, sweating, rapid heart beat, avoidance behavior, and difficulty breathing. Most phobic individuals are aware of the irrationality of their fear, and many endure intense anxiety rather than disclose their disorder. Simple phobias are among the most common medical disorders; in many mild cases, however, they are not significant enough to require treatment.

Obsessive-Compulsive Disorder Symptoms

Obsessive-compulsive disorder (OCD) has been described as hiccups of the mind. Obsessions are recurrent or persistent mental images, thoughts, or ideas, which may result in compulsive behaviors, repetitive, rigid, and self-prescribed routines that are intended to prevent the manifestation of the obsession. It often co-exists with depression and anxiety. Although individuals recognize that the obsessive thoughts and ritualized behavior patterns are senseless and excessive, they cannot stop them in spite of strenuous efforts to ignore or suppress the thoughts or actions. Obsessions and compulsions do not always coexist; however, over half of OCD sufferers have obsessive thoughts without ritualistic behavior. There is some evidence that the symptoms improve over time and that nearly half will eventually recover completely or have only minor symptoms.

OCD is time-consuming, distressing, and can disrupt normal functioning. Much research suggests that a critical feature in this disorder is an over-inflated sense of responsibility, in which the patient's thoughts center around possible dangers and an urgent need to do something about it. The obsessive thoughts or images can range from mundane worries about whether one has locked a door to bizarre and frightening fantasies of behaving violently toward a loved one. The compulsive acts triggered by such obsessions might include repetitive checking for locked doors or unlit stove burners or calls to loved ones at frequent intervals to be sure they are safe. Some people are compelled to wash their hands every few minutes or spend inordinate amounts of time cleaning their surroundings in order to subdue the fear of contagion. Certain other obsessive disorders, including body dysmorphic disorder (BDD), trichotillomania, and Tourette's syndrome, may be part of the OCD spectrum. In BDD, people are obsessed with the belief that they are extremely ugly. People with trichotillomania continually pull their hair, leaving bald patches. Symptoms of Tourette's syndrome include jerky movements, tics, and uncontrollably uttering obscene words. OCD should not be confused with obsessive-compulsive personality, which defines certain character traits (e.g., being a perfectionist, excessively consciousness, morally rigid, and preoccupied with rules and order). These traits do not necessarily occur in people with obsessive-compulsive disorder, which is a psychiatric condition.

Post-Traumatic Stress Disorder Symptoms

Post-traumatic stress disorder (PTSD) is an extreme and usually chronic emotional reaction to a traumatic event that severely impairs ones life; it is classified as an anxiety disorder because of the similarity of symptoms.

Triggering Events. PTSD is triggered by events that are usually thought to be outside the norm of human experience. Such events include, but are not limited to, experiencing or even witnessing sexual assaults, accidents, combat, or unexpected deaths in loved ones. PTSD may also occur in people who have serious illness and receive aggressive treatments or who have close family members or friends with such conditions.

Acute Stress Disorder. Experts have identified a syndrome called acute stress disorder, which occurs within two days to four weeks after the traumatic event, and can help predict who is at highest risk for PTSD. To be diagnosed with acute stress disorder, victims should meet these criteria:

1. They are exposed to traumatic events in which they witness or have been confronted by an actual or potential threat of death, serious injury, or physical harm (such as rape) to themselves or others.

2. Their response is one of fear, helplessness, or horror. In addition, during or after these experiences, they must have three or more of the following symptoms, which indicate a psychological state known as dissociation: an emotional numbness, being in a daze, a sense of losing contact with external reality, a feeling of loss of self or identity, or inability to remember important aspects of the event.

3. They persistently re-experience the trauma in at least one of the following ways: in recurrent images, thoughts, flashbacks, dreams, or feelings of distress at situations that remind them of the traumatic event.

4. They avoid reminders of the event, such as thoughts, people, or any other factors that trigger recollection.

5. They have symptoms of anxiety or heightened awareness of danger (sleeplessness, irritability, being easily startled, or becoming overly vigilant to unknown dangers).

6. The emotional state significantly impairs normal function and relationships, and they fail to seek necessary help.

7. The condition occurs within four weeks of the event and lasts for at least two days and up to four weeks.

8. The condition is not due to alcohol, medications, or drugs and is not an intensification of a pre-existing psychologic disorder.

The criteria for acute stress disorder are accurate at identifying up to 94% of victims at risk, although between 50% and 80% actually develop PTSD. In other words, it is very sensitive for identification of those at highest danger for

PTSD and less successful in determining specifically who will or will not recover emotionally.

Symptoms Of PTSD Itself. The symptoms of PTSD are similar to those of acute stress syndrome but they last beyond a month and are much more severe, chronic (three months or more), or both. They can also occur months or even years after the traumatic event. Children may engage in play or actions in which the events are repetitively enacted. Other symptoms of PTSD may include emotional withdrawal, phobic avoidance of reminders of the trauma that become severe enough to impair personal and work relationships, hopelessness, self-destructive behavior, personality changes, mood swings, difficulty with sleep, anxiety disorders, and guilt over surviving the event.

What Causes Anxiety Disorders?

A person's genetics, biochemistry, environment, and psychologic profile all seem to contribute to the development of anxiety disorders. Most people with these disorders seem to have a biological vulnerability to stress, making them more susceptible to environmental stimuli than the normal population.

✤ **It's A Fact!!**

An estimated 20–25% of close relatives of people with panic disorder or obsessive-compulsive disorder also experience panic or obsessive-compulsive disorders.

Biochemical Factors

Abnormalities In The Brain. Studies suggest that an imbalance of certain substances called neurotransmitters (chemical messengers in the brain) may contribute to anxiety disorders. Advanced imaging techniques have revealed over-activity in the locus ceruleus, the part of the brain important in triggering a response to danger, in people experiencing anxiety, indicating that some people's brains may be more vulnerable to the disorder. Scientists are now beginning to identify different areas of the brain associated with anxiety responses. For example, scans using magnetic resonance imaging techniques of people with OCD, generalized anxiety, and panic disorder have detected abnormalities in the amygdala, a part of the brain that regulates fear, memory, and emotion and coordinates them with heart rate, blood pressure, and other physical responses to stressful events. Abnormalities in a pathway of nerves, referred to as the basal-ganglia thalamocortical pathway, have been linked to OCD, attention deficit disorder, and Tourette's syndrome. The symptoms of the three disorders are similar and they often coexist.

Genetic Factors. About 20% to 25% of close relatives of people with panic disorder or obsessive-compulsive disorder experience these disorders. Researchers have identified a gene associated with people who have personality traits that include anxiety, anger, hostility, impulsiveness, pessimism, and depression. The gene produces reduced amounts of a protein that transports serotonin, an important neurotransmitter for maintaining positive emotions. (This gene, however, would account for only a very small fraction of people with anxiety disorders.) Genetic mutations that affect other neurotransmitters have also been identified that contribute to obsessive-compulsive disorder. The importance of genetics in GAD is still being investigated. Some experts have identified a genetic defect that affects dopamine, another important neurotransmitter, which appears to cause a syndrome that includes migraine headaches, anxiety, and depression.

Family Dynamics

The influence of the family on anxiety is complicated by both genetic and psychologic factors. Many patients with anxiety disorders appear to report parents who were at once overprotective and unaffectionate. One recent study suggested that stressful events, such as disagreements with parents, act upon internalized emotions in young adolescents; eventually these feelings build up and produce full-blown anxiety or depression disorders in young adulthood.

Panic Disorder And Family Influence. Psychodynamic theories suggest that panic disorder is caused by the inability to solve the early childhood conflict of dependence vs. independence. (This theory is backed up by one study reporting that young adults who had experienced childhood anxiety were more likely to live with their parents until their early to mid-twenties.) Many people with panic disorder perceive their parents as being extremely controlling and overly protective while showing little affection.

Phobias And Family Influence. Several studies show a strong correlation between a parent's fears and those of the offspring. Although an inherited trait may be present, some researchers believe that many children can even "learn" fears and phobias just by observing a parent or loved one's phobic or fearful reaction to an event. People who have severe agoraphobia with or without panic disorder generally report less parental affection and more strictness, overprotection, and encouragement of dependence than those without these disorders.

Obsessive Compulsive Disorder And Family Influence. One study found that parental influence played no part in obsessive-compulsive disorder if the patient was also not suffering from depression. (Patients who had both OCD and depression reported lower levels of parental care and over-protectiveness.) It should be noted, however, that the depression coexists in two-thirds of OCD patients.

Traumatic Events

Traumatic events can trigger anxiety disorders, the most obvious being post-traumatic stress syndrome, although there usually needs to be other factors that make one susceptible to anxiety afterward. Specific traumatic events in childhood, however, including abuse—sexual, physical, or both— can cause anxiety and other emotional disorders later on. Some individuals may even have a biological propensity for specific fears, for instance of spiders or snakes, that can be triggered and perpetuated after a single first exposure.

Chemical Hypersensitivity

Some people have panic attacks after exposure to certain foods or chemicals, such as those contained in perfumes or hair sprays. Some studies have indicated that many children and adults with anxiety disorders may have a hypersensitive response to high levels of carbon dioxide, which can occur in crowded spaces, such as airplanes or elevators.

Other Factors

Anxiety can be a chronic symptom of other psychologic or medical problems, such as depression, substance abuse, or thyroid disease. A number of studies have reported a strong link between childhood rheumatic fever, which is caused by a streptococcal infection, and the development of tic-related disorders, including OCD and Tourette's syndrome. The effects of alcohol on the developing fetus now appear to increase the risk for mental disorders as well as birth defects.

❖ **It's A Fact!!**

According to one study, depression in adolescence was a strong predictor of risk for developing generalized anxiety disorder (GAD) in adulthood.

Who Gets Anxiety Disorders?

Age

Anxiety disorders affect more than 23 million Americans, and as many as 25% of all American adults experience intense anxiety at sometime in their lives. The prevalence of severe anxiety disorders is much lower, however. For example, studies indicate that the prevalence of panic disorder among adults is between 1.6% and 2%. It may be much higher in adolescents, however, with studies reporting a prevalence of 3.5% to 9%. Worry is very common among children and is often intense, but only about 5% have anxiety that can be classified as a disorder; moreover, depression is a common companion in such children. Studies have suggested that extremely shy children and those likely to be the target of bullies are at higher risk for developing anxiety disorders later in life. One study suggests that such children could be identified as early as two years of age and possibly treated to avoid later anxiety disorders. Although panic disorders tend to begin in late adolescence and peak at around 25 years of age, in one study, 18% of adult patients with panic disorder reported the onset of the disorder before 10 years of age. Signs of obsessive-compulsive disorder (OCD) can occur in childhood but usually develop fully in adulthood. The risk for generalized anxiety disorder spans a lifetime although it appears to be the most common form of anxiety at older ages. One study reported that depression in adolescence was a strong predictor of generalized anxiety disorder (GAD) in adulthood. The onset of social anxiety disorder usually occurs in adolescence, although most people with this disorder are not diagnosed and do not receive treatment until or unless they develop an accompanying anxiety disorder.

Gender

Women have twice the risk for most anxiety disorders that men do, although obsessive-compulsive disorder occurs equally in both genders. A number of factors may increase the risk in women, including hormonal factors, cultural pressures to meet everyone else's needs except their own, and less self-restrictions on reporting anxiety to physicians. The effects of pregnancy on panic disorder appear to be mixed; it seems to improve the condition in some women and worsen it in others. Like other anxiety disorders, the rates of social phobia are higher in women. Men are more likely than women to seek treatment for this disorder, however (unlike their response to other emotional disorders), probably because social phobias can interfere strongly with many jobs in white-collar professions.

Family History

Anxiety disorders run in families. Although family dynamics and psychologic influences are often at work, genetic factors may also play a role in many cases.

Socioeconomic Factors

A study of Mexican adults living in California reported that native-born Mexican-Americans were three times more likely to have anxiety disorders (and even more likely to be depressed) as those who had recently immigrated to America. And the longer the immigrants lived in the US the greater was their risk for psychiatric problems. Traditional Mexican cultural effects and social ties, then, appear to protect newly arrived immigrants from mental illness, even when they are poor. Eventually, however, the consequences of Americanization lead to depression and anxiety, probably resulting from feelings of alienation and inferiority, not only in many Mexican Americans, but in other impoverished minority groups.

Risk Factors For Post-Traumatic Stress Disorder

Nationwide PTSD affects about 0.8% of men and 1.2% of women, but in specific groups, such as combat troops, the risk is much higher. Among adolescents, studies have found the prevalence of PTSD to be as high as 8.1%. Simply experiencing a traumatic event does not predict post-traumatic stress disorder. Studies estimated that between 6% to 30% or more of trauma survivors develop PTSD, with children being among those at the high end of the range. In a study of individuals who had suffered physical or sexual abuse or neglect as children, about a third developed PTSD. Most did not; negative family or other influences in addition to the traumatic conditions contributed to the risk for this disorder. A number of factors increase vulnerability to catastrophic events, including having a psychiatric illness, drug or alcohol abuse, a family history of anxiety, a history of physical or sexual abuse (particularly violent assaults), and an early separation from parents. One study reported that having a pre-existing emotional disorder, particularly depression, before the traumatic event most often predicted PTSD in women.

How Serious Are Anxiety Disorders?

Association With Depression And Increased Risk For Suicide

Anxiety and depression often go hand and hand. For example, studies have reported that between 20% and 75% of people with panic attacks also have major depression. More than two-thirds of OCD patients also suffer from depression. In a recent report, over half of patients with depression met the criteria for anxiety disorders. Generalized anxiety disorder and social phobia were more likely to precede depression while panic disorder and ago-

> ✤ **It's A Fact!!**
> One study reported that panic attacks were a risk factor for suicide attempts in 13 and 14 year olds.

raphobia were more likely to follow depression. The combination is a risk factor for both substance abuse and suicide. Although suicidal patients with anxiety disorders also often have major depression, a recent study on suicide attempts in young adolescents 13 to 14 years old reported that panic attacks were a risk factor even if depression was not present. Other studies report that 25% to 30% of people with panic disorder harbor suicidal thoughts at some point. Studies have also reported that 18% of people with panic disorder, 12% of those with social phobias, and 13% of patients with OCD had attempted suicide. A number of studies have reported a high association between suicide attempts and panic attacks even in adolescents.

Effects On Physical Health

People with panic disorder perceive their own physical and emotional well being as poor and seek medical help more often than do those in the general population. Studies, in fact, have reported that between 25% and 60% of patients with chest pain who see a physician for possible heart problems suffer instead from panic disorder. Any causal connection between anxiety and medical disorders is unclear. Although a 1998 study found no association between coronary artery disease and anxiety in either men or women, anxiety itself may trigger acute events, such as asthma or chest pain. In fact, panic disorders and phobias have been associated with a higher rate of sudden death from cardiac events. Some researchers speculate that intense anxiety might trigger an abnormal and dangerous heart rhythm, called ventricular fibrillation. Another study indicated that people who experience anxiety are more likely to develop high blood pressure than are those who are not anxious. Both anxiety and depression have been associated with a poor response to treatment in heart patients. Anxiety frequently accompanies medical conditions; for example, half the cases of irritable bowel syndrome are related to anxiety. One study reported that 32% of people with chronic tension headaches met criteria for anxiety; it isn't clear whether the psychologic disorder preceded or followed the onset of headaches. Similarly, another study reported that young girls with anxiety disorder were three times more likely to have chronic headaches than those without the disorder. (Headaches in both these studies were also strongly associated with depression.) No hard evidence exists, however, that anxiety causes these physical problems or that treating anxiety alone will benefit the patient's physical health.

People with obsessive-compulsive disorders can experience skin problems from excessive washing, injuries from repetitive physical acts, and hair loss from repeated hair-pulling, a specific OCD known as trichotillomania.

Alcoholism And Substance Abuse

Severely depressed or anxious people are at high risk for alcoholism, smoking, and other forms of addiction. Anxiety disorders are highly prevalent among people with alcoholism. Among the anxiety disorders, social phobia appears to pose a particular risk for alcoholism. (Specific phobias, interestingly, do not.) One study suggested alcohol itself, however, has no direct beneficial effect on anxiety but that many believe it does. In the study, one group of individuals with social phobia were led to believe they were drinking alcohol (but were not). They experienced less stage fright than those who knew they were not drinking alcohol. Self-medicating anxiety with alcohol, then, has to do with the belief in its benefits rather than any true chemical effects. It should be noted, moreover, that long-term alcohol use can itself cause biologic changes that may actually produce anxiety and depression.

Effects On Work And Relationships

In one study, nearly half of those who suffered from psychiatric disorders before or during their first marriage were divorced compared to a divorce rate of 36% in those who those who never suffered from emotional disorders. Anxiety can also have a negative impact on work. In one survey of OCD sufferers, for example, 40% reported that they had to stop working because of the disorder; only 40% worked full-time, and only half were married.

Outlook For Post-Traumatic Stress Disorder

The long-term impact of a traumatic event is uncertain. In one study of people who survived a mass killing spree in Texas, less than half of those who suffered PTSD (28% of all survivors) had recovered after a year. Survivors of natural catastrophes, such as earthquakes and hurricanes, appear to have an impaired immune response, which may cause problems over time. Some studies on people, including military veterans, who have endured major traumatic events have found a higher risk for health problems. A recent study of Vietnam veterans reported that PTSD was associated with greater physical limitations, poorer physical health, and a lower quality of life than in those in the normal population, regardless of other accompanying emotional or medical disorders. One study of twins, however, reported that among those who had served in Vietnam, combat stress increased some hearing and skin problems but had no major impact on health. According to two new studies, there is growing evidence that heavy smoking and substance abuse are prevalent in people with PTSD, however more studies are needed before an association between PTSD and substance abuse can be determined. Certainly PTSD in adolescence increases the risk for drugs, alcohol, and eating disorders. Of additional concern is a recent study reporting that most adolescents at risk for PTSD are not treated. PTSD may cause actual physical changes in the brain. Two studies reported that Vietnam veterans and women with PTSD who had been sexually abused displayed a 7% to 8% shrinkage in the hippocampus, the part of the brain important for memory and learning. Studies of animals indicate that such damage may result from long term exposure to cortisol, the major stress hormone. Groups who had suffered severe trauma also scored 40% lower in tests of verbal memory than the general population. There was no difference in IQ or in scores of other types of memory.

What Will Confirm A Diagnosis Of An Anxiety Disorder?

Physical Examination And History

Because anxiety accompanies so many medical conditions, some serious, it is extremely important for the physician to uncover any medical problems or medications that might underlie or be masked by an anxiety attack. A physical examination and medical and personal history is essential. The patient should describe any occurrence of anxiety disorders or depression in the family and mention any other contributing factors, such as excessive caffeine use, recent life changes, or stressful events. It is very important to be honest with the physician about all conditions, including excessive drinking, substance abuse, or other psychologic or mood states, that might contribute to or result from the anxiety disorder. Post-traumatic stress disorder (PTSD) is often improperly diagnosed; reasons for this include a high rate of another accompanying disorder that may mask PTSD, patient denial, or failure by the physician to ask about any history of trauma. Standard medical criteria for PTSD may also be too strict, and individuals who actually have the condition may be missed by many physicians.

Other Conditions That Accompany Or Resemble Anxiety Disorders

Anxiety attacks can mimic or accompany nearly every acute disorder of the heart or lungs, including heart attacks and angina. One study reported that 25% of patients entering the emergency room with chest pain were actually suffering from panic attacks, which were diagnosed correctly by

❖ It's A Fact!!
Anxiety Disorders In Adolescents: A Self-Test

How much stress or worry is considered too much? Complete the following self-test by answering "yes" or "no" to the following questions and reviewing the results with your health care professional.

Yes or no? As an teenager are you troubled by:

- Repeated, unexpected "attacks" during which you suddenly are overcome by intense fear or discomfort for no apparent reason, or the fear of having another panic attack?

- Persistent, inappropriate thoughts, impulses or images that you can't get out of your mind (such as a preoccupation with getting dirty or worry about the order of things)?

- Distinct and ongoing fear of social situations involving unfamiliar people?

- Excessive worrying about a number of events or activities?

- Fear of places or situations where getting help or escape might be difficult, such as in a crowd or on an elevator?

- Shortness of breath or a racing heart for no apparent reason?

- Persistent and unreasonable fear of an object or situation, such as flying, heights, animals, blood, etc.?

- Being unable to travel alone, without a companion?

- Spending too much time each day doing things over and over again (for example, hand washing, checking things, or counting)?

cardiologists in only 2% of cases. It is often difficult to distinguish between a heart condition and a panic attack. Mitral valve prolapse, a common and usually mild heart problem, may have symptoms that are nearly identical to those of panic disorder and the two conditions frequently occur together. Two-thirds of people with a heart-rhythm disturbance called paroxysmal supraventricular tachycardia have the same symptoms as those with panic attacks. Women who are having actual heart events are much more likely to

More days than not, do you:

- Feel restless?
- Feel easily fatigued or distracted?
- Experience muscle tension or problem sleeping?

More days than not, do you feel:

- Sad or depressed?
- Disinterested in life?
- Worthless or guilty?

Other questions to consider:

- Have you experienced changes in sleeping or eating habits?
- Do you relive a traumatic event through thoughts, games, distressing dreams, or flashbacks?
- Does your anxiety interfere with your daily life?

Reference

- *Diagnostic and Statistical Manual of Mental Disorders, Fourth Edition.* Washington, DC, American Psychiatric Association, 1994.

Source: Anxiety Disorders Association of America, 1190 Parklawn Drive, Suite 100, Rockville, MD 20852, USA. Reproduced with permission of the Anxiety Disorders Association of America.

be misdiagnosed as having an anxiety attack than men with similar problems. Asthma attacks and panic attacks have similar symptoms and can also coexist. In addition, anxiety-like symptoms are seen in many other medical problems, including epilepsy, hypoglycemia, adrenal-gland tumors, and hyperthyroidism. Women can also experience intense anxiety attacks with hot flashes during menopause.

Many drugs, including some for high blood pressure, diabetes, and thyroid disorders, can produce symptoms of anxiety. Withdrawal from certain drugs, often those used to treat sleep disorders or anxiety, can also precipitate anxiety reactions.

Overuse of caffeine or abuse of amphetamines can cause symptoms resembling a panic attack. People with anxiety disorders often drink alcohol or abuse drugs in order to conceal or ameliorate symptoms, but substance abuse and dependency can also cause anxiety. In addition, withdrawal from alcohol can produce physiologic symptoms similar to panic attacks. Clinicians often have difficulty determining whether alcoholism or anxiety is the primary disorder.

Depression affects as many as 40% of patients with panic disorder. It is sometimes difficult to distinguish from anxiety disorders because depression is often accompanied by anxious feelings, agitation, insomnia, and problems with concentration. (Because of the confusion in making a diagnosis between the two disorders, the American Psychiatric Association is considering a new classification, mixed anxiety and depression.)

Diagnostic Tests

Although most family physicians can identify panic disorder, very few (10% in one study) recognize social phobias. Clinicians can use various tests to determine the causes, type, severity, and frequency of anxiety. Such tests include the Beck Anxiety Inventory, a self-administered test, the Hamilton Anxiety Rating Scale, and the Anxiety Disorders Interview Schedule.

It is also possible to detect correlates of anxiety by assessment of the autonomic nervous system functions, for example heart rate, blood pressure, muscle tension, and respiratory rate. These measurements can help gauge the severity of a person's anxiety.

What Are The General Guidelines For Treating Anxiety Disorders?

Treatment Options

Anxiety disorders require treatment; simply trying to talk oneself out of anxiety is as futile as trying to talk oneself out of a heart or stomach problem. Most anxiety disorders, especially the phobias, respond well to treatment. Combining medications, typically antidepressants known as SSRIs, with cognitive-behavioral therapies (CBT), is proving to be the best treatment options for panic disorders, phobias, including performance anxiety, and even obsessive-compulsive disorder (OCD). Post-traumatic stress disorder (PTSD) is particularly hard to treat, but specific behavioral approaches in the early stages of PTSD are showing promise.

Table 21.1. Treatments for Anxiety Disorders

Anxiety Disorder	Drug Treatment Options	Cognitive-Behavioral and other Non-Drug Therapies
Generalized Anxiety Disorder	Benzodiazepines; buspirone; tricyclics (TCAs) for patients who also are depressed.	Cognitive-behavioral, interpersonal therapy, stress management, biofeedback
Panic Attacks	SSRIs; benzodiazepines; TCAs, MAO inhibitors.	Cognitive-behavioral therapy
Phobias	Benzodiazepines; beta-blockers; SSRIs.	Cognitive-behavioral therapy (desensitization therapy), hypnosis
Obsessive-Compulsive Disorder	SSRIs as first choice, except if tics are present (neuroleptics for tics); clomipramine (a tricyclic); MAO inhibitors for those who do not respond to other drugs.	Cognitive-behavioral therapy (Exposure and response prevention)
Post-traumatic Stress Disorder	Antidepressants, clonidine	Cognitive-behavioral therapy (Group therapy).

Note: For anxiety disorders, the most effective treatments are usually combinations of drugs and behavioral techniques.

Life Style Measures

A healthy lifestyle that includes exercise, adequate rest, and good nutrition can help to reduce the impact of anxiety attacks. Rhythmic aerobic and yoga exercise programs lasting for more than 15 weeks have been found to help reduce anxiety. Strength, or resistance, training does not seem to help anxiety.

What Medications Are Used For Anxiety Disorder?

Until recently, the anti-anxiety drugs known as benzodiazepines were the primary medications for anxiety. Increasingly, antidepressants, particularly the selective serotonin-reuptake inhibitors (SSRIs), are being used as the initial treatment. They are proving to be effective, nonaddictive, and to have relatively minor side effects than the standard anti-anxiety drugs known as benzodiazapines. It should noted that one problem with their use is that many standard antidepressants require a long delay before they are fully effective, usually two to four weeks, and sometimes up to 12 weeks. People who take them may also experience a temporary period of increased anxiety. Consequently, about a third of patients stop taking antidepressants for anxiety disorders before the initial phase of therapy has been completed. A combination of a benzodiazapine and an antidepressant then is sometimes used to avoid the initial anxiety symptoms and to hasten control of panic symptoms. No one should give up if one drug treatment fails; another may prove to be very effective, even it is a drug of a similar type. Drug combinations should be tried generally only if a single drug and cognitive-behavior therapy have failed. Because many anxiety disorders are chronic, drug therapy sometimes is needed for prolonged periods, even years.

Antidepressants

Selective Serotonin Reuptake Inhibitors (SSRIs). Fluoxetine (Prozac), sertraline (Zoloft), paroxetine (Paxil), citalopram (Celexa), and fluvoxamine (Luvox) are antidepressant drugs known as selective serotonin reuptake inhibitors (SSRIs). They are recommended as the first line of treatment for obsessive-compulsive disorder, and appear to reduce symptoms by 25% to 35% in about half of all patients. Low-dose maintenance therapy may be sufficient for patients who respond well to initial therapy, although most patients do not have a fully adequate response; they require high doses. People with OCD and hoarding or compulsive behaviors may not respond as well to SSRIs as do those without these symptoms. These antidepressants are also less effective in OCD patients with tics, for whom small doses of drugs known as neuroleptics may be helpful. Both fluvoxamine and sertraline are also beneficial in treating patients with panic disorder and agoraphobia. SSRIs may also be helpful for social phobias, but relapse is common even after prolonged treatment if they are not combined with cognitive-behavioral treatments. Studies have also indicated that fluvoxamine, sertraline, and paroxetine may even help some people with post-traumatic stress disorder (PTSD). (Victims of child abuse tend to respond poorly, whether or not the abuse was the specific trauma triggering PTS.) SSRIs can cause agitation, nausea, and sexual dysfunction, including delay in or loss of orgasm and low sexual drive. (Taking a supervised drug "holiday" on the weekend may improve sexual function during that time, although it may also cause dizziness, exhaustion, and depression.) Some patients, during the first few weeks of treatment, lose a small amount of weight but generally regain it. Elderly people taking these drugs should take the lowest effective dose possible, and those with heart problems should be monitored closely.

Designer Antidepressants. Newer antidepressants are being specifically designed to target mechanisms that elevate serotonin and other neurotransmitters in the brain; some showing promise for anxiety are venlafaxine (Effexor) and nefazodone (Serzone). Mirtazapine (Remeron), a unique antidepressant known as a 5-HT2 blocker, is particularly promising; it may be an effective treatment for panic disorder, generalized anxiety disorder, obsessive-compulsive disorder, and even post-traumatic stress disorder. Compared to some common SSRIs, studies are indicating that it becomes effective more rapidly and has stronger early actions against anxiety in patients who also suffer depression. It also causes less sexual dysfunction than other drugs. It interacts with histamine, a chemical involved in allergic responses; these actions can cause drowsiness, which may make it a useful drug for patients who suffer from insomnia. However, it also causes blurred vision. The drug has been associated with weight gain, although in one study it was not significant. It does not appear to have the adverse acute effects on the heart that other newer antidepressants have, although it may elevate cholesterol and triglyceride levels slightly.

Tricyclic Antidepressants. The antidepressant drugs known as tricyclic antidepressants (TCA) have also been effective in treating panic and obsessive-compulsive disorders. The most common TCA used for the treatment of panic disorder is imipramine (Tofranil, Janimine); it is also effective in treating agoraphobia, including those with panic disorder. For people with a mix of generalized anxiety disorder and depression, doxepin (Adapin, Sinequan) has been beneficial. Clomipramine (Anafranil) is also effective for panic disorders and has been approved for OCD. The drug causes significant reduction in OCD symptoms for patients who can tolerate it, but many patients stop using it because of side effects and even many of those who stay on the drug experience adverse effects. Anafranil has more adverse side effects than the SSRIs; both appear to be equally effective over time. (The other tricyclics do not appear to benefit OCD patients.) Side effects of TCAs include sleep disturbance, abrupt reduction in blood pressure upon standing, weight gain, sexual dysfunction, and mental disturbance. Elderly patients and those with a history of seizures, cardiac problems, closed-angle glaucoma, and urinary retention or obstruction should be closely supervised when taking tricyclics.

Monamine Oxidase Inhibitors. Monoamine oxidase inhibitors (MAOIs), typically phenelzine (Nardil) or tranylcypromine (Parnate), are antidepressants used for panic disorder or OCD that does not respond to other treatments. MAOIs commonly cause weight gain, drowsiness, dizziness, sexual dysfunction, and insomnia. They can also cause birth defects and should not be taken by pregnant women. Hypertension, a potentially serious side effect, can be brought on by eating certain foods, including cheese, red wine, vermouth, dried meats and fish, canned figs, and fava beans, that have a high tyramine content. MAOIs can have serious interactions with certain drugs, including some common over-the-counter cough medications and decongestants. Fatal reactions have occurred when SSRIs and MAOIs were taken at the same time. There should be at least a two to three-week break if a patient is changing from one type of antidepressant to the other. (There should be a five-week break after taking Prozac and before taking an MAOI.)

Benzodiazepines

Benzodiazepines have, until recently, been the standard treatment of most anxiety disorders; these drugs reinforce a chemical in the brain that inhibits nerve-cell excitability. Alprazolam (Xanax) and clonazepam (Klonopin) are effective for panic disorder, agoraphobia, and generalized anxiety disorder. Other benzodiazepines, including diazepam (Valium), lorazepam (Ativan), halazepam (Paxipam), and chlordiazepoxide (Librium), are used mainly for generalized anxiety.

Common side effects of benzodiazepines are daytime drowsiness and a hung-over feeling. Respiratory problems may be exacerbated. The drugs appear to stimulate eating and can cause weight gain. Benzodiazepines can interact with certain drugs, including cimetidine (Tagamet) and antihistamines. Benzodiazepines are potentially dangerous when used in combination with alcohol. Overdoses are serious, although very rarely fatal. Elderly people are more susceptible to side effects and should usually start at half the dose prescribed for younger people. Of great concern are studies showing automobile accidents and a high risk for hip fractures from falls in older people who take benzodiazepines. They are associated with birth defects, and should not be used by pregnant women or nursing mothers.

The primary problem with these drugs is their loss of effectiveness over time with continued use at the same dosage. As a result, patients may require increasing doses to prevent anxiety. Dependence is a common danger, which can occur after as short a time as three months. People who discontinue benzodiazepines after taking them for long periods may experience rebound symptoms, sleep disturbance, and anxiety, which can develop within hours or days after stopping the medication. Some patients experience withdrawal symptoms, including stomach distress, sweating, and insomnia, that can last from one to three weeks.

Azapirones

Buspirone (BuSpar) is an azapirone, a class of drugs showing promise for generalized anxiety disorder. Unfortunately, it usually takes several days to weeks for the drug to be fully effective, and it is not useful against panic attacks. Unlike the benzodiazepines, buspirone is not addictive, even with long-term use, and it seems to have less pronounced side effects and no withdrawal effects, even when the drug is discontinued quickly. The drug does not produce any immediate euphoria or change in sensation, so some people believe, erroneously, that the drug doesn't work. Because it has a low potential for abuse, buspirone is useful in persons whose anxiety disorder coexists with alcoholism. Some experts also think it may be useful for adolescents and children. Common side effects include dizziness, drowsiness, and nausea. Patients who have recently been taking benzodiazepines may respond less well to buspirone than others. BuSpar should not be used with monoamine oxidase inhibitors (MAOIs).

Beta-Blockers

Beta-blockers, including propranolol (Inderal) and atenolol (Tenormin), block the nerves that stimulate the heart to beat faster. They affect only the physiologic symptoms of anxiety and are most helpful for phobias, particularly performance anxiety. Beta-blockers are less successful for other forms of anxiety.

Clonidine

Clonidine, a drug that relaxes blood vessels, has been used to treat children with post-traumatic stress disorder. Anxiety was reduced and behavior improved, and some experts believe it should be tried if other therapies fail. The drug can have severe side effects.

Investigative Drugs

Pagoclone is known as a gamma amino butyric acid (GABA) receptor modulator. It is showing promise in trials for significantly reducing panic attacks with few side effects. Substance-P is a brain chemical that is believed to have a role in increasing mood disorders. In one investigative trial of patients with major depression, a substance-P blocker termed MK-869 reduced anxiety as well as depression.

What Are The Psychotherapeutic And Other Non-Drug Approaches To Anxiety Disorder?

Cognitive-Behavioral Therapy

A number of cognitive-behavioral therapeutic (CBT) approaches have been designed to treat both the general symptoms of anxiety and specific disorders. CBT and especially group therapy for children may even help people with post-traumatic stress disorder. CBT works on the principle that the thoughts that produce and maintain anxiety can be recognized objectively and altered using various techniques, thereby changing the behavioral response and eliminating the anxiety reaction. The goal is to regain control of reactions to stress and stimuli, thus reducing the feeling of helplessness that often accompanies anxiety disorders. A small study comparing cognitive therapy with emotional supportive therapy reported that after two months, 70% of those using cognitive therapy, but only 25% of the other group, were free of panic attacks. Treatments are equally effective in men and women. Anxiety disorders are chronic, however, and recurrence is common. Some studies indicate, in fact, that between 30% and 82% of people with panic disorder and phobias have a recurrence of attacks at an average of nine months even after successful short-term therapy. (Women are at much higher risk for recurrence of panic attacks than men.) Medications, then, are also generally recommended for most patients. There may be exceptions. For example, behavioral therapy alone may be as effective as medications for children with OCD.

Basic Cognitive Therapy Techniques. Treatment usually takes about 12 to 20 weeks. First, the patient must learn how to recognize anxious reactions and thoughts as they occur. These entrenched and automatic reactions and thoughts must be challenged and understood. One of the most important steps is to keep a daily diary that reports the occurrences of the anxiety attack and any thoughts and events associated with it. As the patient begins perceiving that false assumptions underlie the anxiety, he or she can begin substituting new ways of coping with the feared objects and situations. The essential goal of cognitive therapy is to understand the realities of an anxiety-provoking situation and to respond to reality with new actions based on reasonable expectations. For example, some cognitive therapists are approaching treatment of OCD patients by seeking to change their ideas about their heightened sense of responsibility for preventing harm. Techniques for OCT may include keeping a diary of repetitive thinking events, using an audio tape to "over-expose" the patient to repetitive thoughts, and self-observation to reduce unrealistic ideas, such as an urgent need to prevent a harmful situation that doesn't exist, and to restructure the thought process. Patients are also usually given behavioral homework assignments; for example, a person with generalized social phobia may be asked to buy an item and then return it the next day, observing as he or she does so the unrealistic fears and thoughts triggered by such an event.

Systematic Desensitization. Systematic desensitization is a specific technique that breaks the link between the anxiety-provoking stimulus and the anxiety response; this treatment requires the patient to gradually confront the object of fear. There are three main elements to the process: relaxation training, a list composed by the patient that prioritizes anxiety-inducing situations by degree of fear, and the desensitization procedure itself—confronting each item on the list, starting with the least stressful. This treatment is especially effective for simple phobias, social phobias, agoraphobia, and post-traumatic stress syndrome.

Exposure And Response Treatment. Exposure treatment purposefully generates anxiety, unlike the desensitization process, which emphasizes a relaxed approach and allows the patient to gradually confront the sources of anxiety. By repeatedly exposing the patient to the feared object or situation, either literally or using imagination, the patient experiences the anxiety over and over until the stimulating event eventually loses its effect. Two variants of exposure treatments are flooding and graduated exposure. Flooding, which exposes the person to the anxiety-producing stimulus for as long as one or two hours, has been helpful for some patients with most types of anxiety disorders. Graduated exposure, which can also be successful, gives the patient a greater degree of control over the length and frequency of exposures. Both types of exposure treatment use the most fearful stimulus first, unlike systematic desensitization, which begins with the least fearful. One study reported that prolonged exposure therapy for motor-vehicle accident survivors with acute stress disorder (early symptoms indicating a risk for post-traumatic stress disorder) was effective in preventing full-flown PTSD, which is extremely difficult to treat. Combining exposure with cognitive therapy may be particularly beneficial. The results of this study are not necessarily applicable to other trauma sufferers, such as rape victims.

Modeling Treatment. Phobias can often be treated successfully with modeling treatment; the patient observes an actor approach an anxiety-producing object or engage in a fear-provoking activity that is similar to the patient's specific problem. The goal is to learn how to behave in comparable circumstances. Either a live or video-taped situation may be used, although the live model is considered to be more effective. So-called "virtual reality" may prove to be a very useful modeling tool. This technology employs computer-generated images and special headgear to realistically simulate a natural environment and allow interaction with it. In one case, a psychologist used virtual reality to cure a woman of arachnophobia (fear of spiders). More research is needed.

Relaxation Techniques And Breathing Retraining. As part of many of the CBT approaches, patients are taught techniques to reduce the physical effects of anxiety. For example, many people with anxiety disorders experience hyperventilation, rapid, tense breathing that expels too much carbon dioxide, resulting in chest pain, dizziness, tingling of the mouth and fingers, muscle cramps, and even fainting. Hyperventilation is one of the primary physical manifestations of panic disorders. By practicing measured, controlled breathing at the onset of a panic attack, patients may be able to prevent full attacks. Relaxation methods, such as learning how to gradually relax all the muscles, may also be helpful.

Other Forms Of Psychotherapy

Other forms of psychotherapy, commonly called "talk" therapies, deal more with childhood roots of anxiety and usually, although not always, require longer treatments. They include interpersonal therapy, supportive psychotherapy, attention intervention, and psychoanalysis. All work is done during the sessions. Some experts believe that such therapies might be more useful for generalized anxiety, which may require more sustained work to process and recover from early traumas and fears.

Surgery

A surgical technique called cingulotomy involves interrupting the cingulate gyrus, a bundle of nerve fibers in the front of the brain. It is sometimes used as a last resort for patients with severe OCD. A recent variation of this procedure using magnetic resonance imaging (MRI) to guide the surgeon is resulting in long-term improvement in about one-quarter to one-third of

OCD patients in whom it is performed. The procedure is generally safe with few serious complications and does not affect intellect or memory.

☞ Remember!!

Anxiety disorders are usually caused by a combination of psychological, physical, and genetic conditions, and treatment is, in general, very effective.

Chapter 22

Generalized Anxiety Disorder

Generalized Anxiety Disorder (GAD) is characterized by 6 months or more of chronic, exaggerated worry and tension that is unfounded or much more severe than the normal anxiety most people experience. People with this disorder usually expect the worst; they worry excessively about money, health, family, or work, even when there are no signs of trouble. They are unable to relax and often suffer from insomnia. Many people with GAD also have physical symptoms, such as fatigue, trembling, muscle tension, headaches, irritability, or hot flashes. Fortunately, through research supported by the National Institute of Mental Health (NIMH), effective treatments have been developed to help people with GAD.

How Common Is GAD?

- About 3 to 4% of the U.S. population has GAD during the course of a year.

- GAD most often strikes people in childhood or adolescence, but can begin in adulthood, too. It affects women more often than men.

About This Chapter: The information in this chapter is from "Quick Facts About Generalized Anxiety Disorder," an undated fact sheet produced by the National Institute of Mental Health.

What Causes GAD?

Some research suggests that GAD may run in families, and it may also grow worse during stress. GAD usually begins at an earlier age and symptoms may manifest themselves more slowly than in most other anxiety disorders.

✎ Weird Words

Anxiety: A sense of apprehension and fear often marked by physical symptoms (such as sweating, tension, and increased heart rate).

Anxiolytics: The medications that reduce the symptoms of anxiety.

Behavior therapy: The treatment used to help patients substitute desirable responses and behavior patterns for undesirable ones.

Benzodiazepines: A class of drugs that act as tranquilizers; the most common side effects are drowsiness and withdrawal symptoms upon abrupt ending of treatment.

Cognitive Therapy: A form of therapy stemming from the belief that emotional disorders are caused by irrational yet habitual forms of thinking; these patterns are viewed as behaviors that the therapist can try to help the patient change.

Generalized Anxiety Disorder (GAD): An excessive or unrealistic worry that is unrelated to another illness and can last six months or more.

Progressive Muscle Relaxation: Tensing and relaxing the various muscle groups of the body in a systematic manner, such as starting with the feet and legs and proceeding up the body; this technique has been known to ease generalized anxiety disorder symptoms.

Source: These definitions are excerpted from the Anxiety Disorders Association of America's Glossary on their website at www.adaa.org © 2001. Reproduced with permission of the Anxiety Disorders Association of America.

What Treatments Are Available For GAD?

Treatments for GAD include medications, cognitive-behavioral therapy, relaxation techniques, and biofeedback to control muscle tension. Successful treatment may include a medication called buspirone. Research into the effectiveness of other medications, such as benzodiazapines and antidepressants, is ongoing.

Can People With GAD Also Have Other Physical And Emotional Illnesses?

Research shows that GAD often coexists with depression, substance abuse, or other anxiety disorders. Other conditions associated with stress, such as irritable bowel syndrome, often accompany GAD. Patients with physical symptoms such as insomnia or headaches should also tell their doctors about their feelings of worry and tension. This will help the patient's health care provider to recognize that the person is suffering from GAD.

Chapter 23

Panic Disorder

Panic disorder is a serious condition that may affect about one out of every 75 people. It usually appears during the teens or early adulthood, and while the exact causes are unclear, there does seem to be a connection with major life transitions that are potentially stressful: graduating from college, getting married, having a first child, and so on. There is also some evidence for a genetic predisposition; if a family member has suffered from panic disorder, you have an increased risk of suffering from it yourself, especially during a time in your life that is particularly stressful.

Panic Attacks: The Hallmark Of Panic Disorder

A panic attack is a sudden surge of overwhelming fear that comes without warning and without any obvious reason. It is far more intense than the feeling of being 'stressed out' that most people experience. Symptoms of a panic attack include:

- Racing heartbeat
- Difficulty breathing, feeling as though you 'can't get enough air'
- Terror that is almost paralyzing
- Dizziness, lightheadedness or nausea

About This Chapter: The text in this chapter is from "Answers to Your Questions about Panic Disorder," © 2000 by the American Psychological Association. Reprinted with permission.

- Trembling, sweating, shaking
- Choking, chest pains
- Hot flashes, or sudden chills
- Tingling in fingers or toes ('pins and needles')
- Fear that you're going to go crazy or are about to die

♣ It's A Fact!!

Although panic disorder affects an estimated 1 out of every 75 people, getting a correct diagnosis can be difficult. One study found that people sometimes see 10 or more doctors before being properly diagnosed.

You probably recognize this as the classic 'flight or fight' response that human beings experience when we are in a situation of danger. But during a panic attack, these symptoms seem to rise from out of nowhere. They occur in seemingly harmless situations—they can even happen while you are asleep.

In addition to the above symptoms, a panic attack is marked by the following conditions:

- It occurs suddenly, without any warning and without any way to stop it.
- The level of fear is way out of proportion to the actual situation; often, in fact, it's completely unrelated.
- It passes in a few minutes; the body cannot sustain the 'fight or flight' response for longer than that. However, repeated attacks can continue to recur for hours.

A panic attack is not dangerous, but it can be terrifying, largely because it feels 'crazy' and 'out of control.' Panic disorder is frightening because of the panic attacks associated with it, and also because it often leads to other complications such as phobias, depression, substance abuse, medical complications, even suicide. Its effects can range from mild word or social impairment to a total inability to face the outside world.

In fact, the phobias that people with panic disorder develop do not come from fears of actual objects or events, but rather from fear of having another attack. In these cases, people will avoid certain objects or situations because they fear that these things will trigger another attack.

How To Identify Panic Disorder

Please remember that only a licensed therapist can diagnose a panic disorder. There are certain signs you may already be aware of, though.

One study found that people sometimes see 10 or more doctors before being properly diagnosed, and that only one out of four people with the disorder receive the treatment they need. That's why it's important to know what the symptoms are, and to make sure you get the right help.

Many people experience occasional panic attacks, and if you have had one or two such attacks, there probably isn't any reason to worry. The key symptom of panic disorder is the persistent fear of having future panic attacks. If you suffer from repeated (four or more) panic attacks, and especially if you have had a panic attack and are in continued fear of having another, these are signs that you should consider finding a mental health professional who specializes in panic or anxiety disorders.

What Causes Panic Disorder: Mind, Body, Or Both?

Body

There may be a genetic predisposition to anxiety disorders; some sufferers report that a family member has or had a panic disorder or some other emotional disorder such as depression. Studies with twins have confirmed the possibility of 'genetic inheritance' of the disorder.

Panic Disorder could also be due to a biological malfunction, although a specific biological marker has yet to be identified.

All ethnic groups are vulnerable to panic disorder. For unknown reasons, women are twice as likely to get the disorder as men.

Mind

Stressful life events can trigger panic disorders. One association that has been noted is that of a recent loss or separation. Some researchers liken the 'life stressor' to a thermostat; that is, when stresses lower your resistance, the underlying physical predisposition kicks in and triggers an attack.

✔ Quick Tip

How To Stop A Panic Attack

"Make it stop!" is the battle cry of panic sufferers everywhere. When you feel a panic attack coming on, take these steps.

1. STOP!

People in the midst of a panic attack immediately freak out. "Oh my God, I'm having a heart attack!" "This is it. I'm dying." "I am finally losing my mind."

STOP! Say the word out loud. Put your hands out in front of you and tell yourself, tell your panic, "STOP!"

2. REFOCUS

Once you have reigned in your racing thoughts, divert your attention to an external object or choose a repetitive activity or external diversion.

External Diversions

- Mow the lawn
- Pull some weeds
- Paint a picture
- Scrub a floor
- Call a friend
- Bathe the dog
- Do sit-ups
- Snap a rubber band that you wear on your wrist

Repetitive Diversions

- Say your ABC's backwards
- Recite the Presidents of the U.S.
- How many U.S. states can you name
- Repeat a prayer (For example, "The Lord's Prayer")
- Take your pulse and count each heartbeat

3. BREATHE

"Hyperventilation raises the pH level in the nerve cells, making them more excitable, and it also tends to activate the fight or flight response," says Reneau Peurifoy, M.A, M.F.C.C. in *Anxiety, Phobias, and Panic.* This causes all of those disturbing symptoms we incorrectly assume are heart attacks, strokes or going crazy.

Many sufferers of panic attacks are not breathing correctly. They many times actually hold their breath when anxious. If you find yourself your yawning or sighing a lot, then you probably are one of those people who holds their breath a lot, without even realizing it! Holding your breath causes the carbon dioxide level to drop, resulting in symptoms of hyperventilation, resulting in a panic attack.

To breathe properly, you must breathe from the diaphragm, not from the upper chest. You can test your breathing style by placing one hand on your chest and one hand on your stomach. Relax and breathe normally. If the hand on your chest moves, you are an upper chest breather—not a good thing, unless you are doing strenuous exercise. A normal breather should find that the hand on the stomach moves. This is normal, resting breathing.

Become aware of your breathing patterns. A normal breathing rate at rest is eight to sixteen breaths per minute. One study of people with panic disorder found an average resting breathing rate of twenty eight breaths per minute!

Remember this mantra: SRB: Stop, refocus, BREATHE! Tape it to your mirror, put it in your wallet, paint it on your bedroom wall.

Information in this section is from "How to Stop a Panic Attack," by Karen Rager, published November 9, 1999, © 1996-2000 Suite101.com, Inc., All rights reserved; reprinted with permission. Available online at http://www.suite101.com/article.cfm/panic_disorder/28333.

Both

Physical and psychological causes of panic disorder work together. Although initially attacks may come out of the blue, eventually the sufferer may actually help bring them on by responding to physical symptoms of an attack.

For example, if a person with panic disorder experiences a racing heartbeat caused by drinking coffee, exercising, or taking a certain medication, they might interpret this as a symptom of an attack and, because of their anxiety, actually bring on the attack. On the other hand, coffee, exercise, and certain medications sometimes do, in fact, cause panic attacks. One of the most frustrating things for the panic sufferer is never knowing how to isolate the different triggers of an attack. That's why the right therapy for panic disorder focuses on all aspects—physical, psychological, and physiological— of the disorder.

✎ Weird Words

Anxiety: An emotional state characterized by apprehension, uneasiness, dread of impending danger, or fear; often accompanied by symptoms such as a rapid heartbeat, agitation, tension, and restlessness.

Panic: Sudden, overwhelming fear or anxiety that is extreme and unreasonable, often accompanied by symptoms such as an increased heart rate, rapid breathing, and sweating.

Panic Attack: A period of intense fear or anxiety accompanied by symptoms such as shortness of breath, heart palpitations, sweating, trembling, chest pain, dizziness, and fear of losing control.

Panic Disorder: A mental disorder characterized by recurring and unpredictable panic attacks.

Systematic Desensitization: A form of behavior therapy in which a patient is gradually exposed to a feared stimulus until the stimulus is tolerated without anxiety. Systematic desensitization is sometimes used in the treatment of phobias.

Can People With Panic Disorder Lead Normal Lives?

The answer to this is a resounding YES—if they receive treatment.

Panic disorder is highly treatable, with a variety of available therapies. These treatments are extremely effective, and most people who have successfully completed treatment can continue to experience situational avoidance or anxiety, and further treatment might be necessary in those cases. Once treated, panic disorder doesn't lead to any permanent complications.

Side Effects Of Panic Disorder

Without treatment, panic disorder can have very serious consequences.

The immediate danger with panic disorder is that it can often lead to a phobia. That's because once you've suffered a panic attack, you may start to avoid situations like the one you were in when the attack occurred.

Many people with panic disorder show 'situational avoidance' associated with their panic attacks. For example, you might have an attack while driving, and start to avoid driving until you develop an actual phobia towards it. In worst case scenarios, people with panic disorder develop agoraphobia—fear of going outdoors—because they believe that by staying inside, they can avoid all situations that might provoke an attack, or where they might not be able to get help. The fear of an attack is so debilitating, they prefer to spend their lives locked inside their homes.

Even if you don't develop these extreme phobias, your quality of life can be severely damaged by untreated panic disorder. A recent study showed that people who suffer from panic disorder:

- are more prone to alcohol and other drug abuse
- have greater risk of attempting suicide
- spend more time in hospital emergency rooms
- spend less time on hobbies, sports and other satisfying activities
- tend to be financially dependent on others
- report feeling emotionally and physically less healthy than non-sufferers
- are afraid of driving more than a few miles away from home

Panic disorders can also have economic effects. For example, a recent study cited the case of a woman who gave up a $40,000 a year job that required travel for one close to home that only paid $14,000 a year. Other sufferers have reported losing their jobs and having to rely on public assistance or family members.

None of this needs to happen. Panic disorder can be treated successfully, and sufferers can go on to lead full and satisfying lives.

How Can Panic Disorder Be Treated?

Most specialists agree that a combination of cognitive and behavioral therapies are the best treatment for panic disorder. Medication might also be appropriate in some cases.

The first part of therapy is largely informational; many people are greatly helped by simply understanding exactly what panic disorder is, and how many others suffer from it. Many people who suffer from panic disorder are worried that their panic attacks mean they're 'going crazy' or that the panic might induce a heart attack. 'Cognitive restructuring' (changing one's way of thinking) helps people replace those thoughts with more realistic, positive ways of viewing the attacks.

Cognitive therapy can help the patient identify possible triggers for the attacks. The trigger in an individual case could be something like a thought, a situation, or something as subtle as a slight change in heartbeat. Once the patient understands that the panic attack is separate and independent of the trigger, that trigger begins to lose some of its power to induce an attack.

The behavioral components of the therapy can consist of what one group of clinicians has termed 'interoceptive exposure.' This is similar to the systematic desensitization used to cure phobias, but what it focuses on is exposure to the actual physical sensations that someone experiences during a panic attack.

People with panic disorder are more afraid of the actual attack than they are of specific objects or events; for instance, their 'fear of flying' is not that the planes will crash but that they will have a panic attack in a place, like a plane, where they can't get to help. Others won't drink coffee or go to an overheated room because they're afraid that these might trigger the physical symptoms of a panic attack.

Interoceptive exposure can help them go through the symptoms of an attack (elevated heart rate, hot flashes, sweating, and so on) in a controlled setting, and teach them that these symptoms need not develop into a full-blown attack. Behavioral therapy is also used to deal with the situational avoidance associated with panic attacks. One very effective treatment for phobias is in vivo exposure, which is in its simplest terms means breaking a fearful situation down into small manageable steps and doing them one at a time until the most difficult level is mastered.

Relaxation techniques can further help someone 'flow through' an attack. These techniques include breathing retraining and positive visualization. Some experts have found that people with panic disorder tend to have slightly higher than average breathing rates, learning to slow this can help someone deal with a panic attack and can also prevent future attacks.

In some cases, medications may also be needed. Anti-anxiety medications may be prescribed, as well as antidepressants, and sometimes even heart medications (such as beta blockers) that are used to control irregular heartbeats.

☞ Remember!!

A panic attack is not dangerous, but it can be terrifying, largely because it feels 'crazy' and 'out of control.' Panic disorder is frightening because of the panic attacks associated with it, and also because it often leads to other complications such as phobias, depression, substance abuse, medical complications, even suicide. Most specialists agree that a combination of cognitive and behavioral therapies are the best treatment for panic disorder. Medication might also be appropriate in some cases. Keep in mind that panic disorder, like any other emotional disorder, isn't something you can either diagnose or cure by yourself. An experienced clinical psychologist or psychiatrist is the most qualified person to make this diagnosis, just as he or she is the most qualified to treat this disorder.

Finally, a support group with others who suffer from panic disorder can be very helpful to some people. It can't take the place of therapy, but it can be a useful adjunct.

If you suffer from panic disorder, these therapies can help you. But you can't do them on your own; all of these treatments must be outlined and prescribed by a psychologist or psychiatrist.

How Long Does Treatment Take?

Much of the success of treatment depends on your willingness to carefully follow the outlined treatment plan. This is often multifaceted, and it won't work overnight, but if you stick with it, you should start to have noticeable improvement within about 10 to 20 weekly sessions. If you continue to follow the program, within one year you will notice a tremendous improvement.

If you are suffering from panic disorder, you should be able to find help in your area. You need to find a licensed psychologist or other mental health professional who specializes in panic or anxiety disorders. There may even be a clinic nearby that specializes in these disorders.

When you speak with a therapist, specify that you think you have panic disorder, and ask about his or her experience treating this disorder.

Keep in mind, though, that panic disorder, like any other emotional disorder, isn't something you can either diagnose or cure by yourself. An experience clinical psychologist or psychiatrist is the most qualified person to make this diagnosis, just as he or she is the most qualified to treat this disorder.

This text is designed to answer your basic questions about panic disorder; a qualified mental health professional will be able to give you more complete information.

Panic disorder does not need to disrupt your life in any way!

About The American Psychological Association

The American Psychological Association (APA) located in Washington, D.C., is the largest scientific and professional organization representing psychology in the United States and is the world's largest association of psychologists. APA's membership includes more than 132,000 practitioners, researchers, educators, consultants and students. Through its divisions in 49 subfields of psychology and affiliations with 58 state and territorial and Canadian provincial associations, APA works to advance psychology as a science, as a profession, and as a means of promoting human welfare.

American Psychological Association
Office of Public Affairs
750 First St., NE
Washington, DC 20002
Toll Free: 800-374-2721
Phone: 202-336-5500
Website: http://www.apa.org

Chapter 24

Phobias

From 50 yards away, you see the animal approaching. Silently it watches you as it slinks ever so much closer with each padded step. Stay calm, you tell yourself. There's nothing to fear.

But suddenly, panic seizes you in a death grip, squeezing the breath out of you and turning your knees to Jell-O. Your heart starts slam-dancing inside your chest, your mouth turns to cotton, and your palms are so sweaty you'd swear they'd sprung a leak. You'd escape this terrifying confrontation, if only you could make your legs work!

Just what is this wild and dangerous animal making you hyperventilate and turning your legs to rubber? A man-eating tiger, hungry for a meal? A lioness bent on protecting her cubs? Guess again. That's Tabby, your neighbor's ordinary house cat, sauntering your way. Ridiculous, right? How can anyone experience so much fear at the sight of such an innocuous animal? If you're one of the thousands who suffer from galeophobia—the fear of cats—or any one of hundreds of other phobias, sheer panic at the appearance of everyday objects, situations or feelings is a regular occurrence.

About This Chapter: Text in this chapter is from "Fighting Phobias: The Things That Go Bump In The Mind," by Lynne L. Hall in *FDA Consumer*, U.S. Food and Drug Administration, March 1997.

✎ Weird Words

Phobia: An abnormal, persistent, irrational fear or dread that causes a state of panic. Examples of some phobias include:

Term:	Fear of:	Term:	Fear of:
Acarophobia	mites or small objects like pins and needles	Chronophobia	time
		Claustrophobia	confined spaces
Acousticophobia	loud sounds	Coitophobia	sexual inter-course
Acrophobia	high places		
Agoraphobia	open spaces and fear of leaving the home environ-ment	Coprophobia	excrement
		Cynophobia	dogs, or fear of rabies
		Dermatophobia	skin disease
		Dextrophobia	objects on the right side
Aichmophobia	being touched by pointed objects		
		Eremophobia	deserted places or being alone
Ailurophobia	cats	Ergasiophobia	fear or abnormal dislike of work
Algophobia	experiencing or witnessing pain		
		Erythrophobia	blushing, the color red
Amaxophobia	riding in a vehicle	Gamophobia	marriage
Androphobia	men	Gynephobia	women
Anthropophobia	human companion-ship	Hamartophobia	error or sin
		Haphephobia	being touched
		Harpaxophobia	robbers
Apiphobia	bees; also called melissophobia	Hedonophobia	pleasure
		Hemophobia	blood, either bleeding or seeing blood
Arachnophobia	spiders		
Astraphobia	lightening or stars	Hodophobia	travel
Bathophobia	depths	Hydrophobia	water; also another name for rabies
Bromidrosiphobia	odors		
Brontophobia	thunder		

Term:	Fear of:	Term:	Fear of:
Hylophobia	the forest	Pathophobia	disease; also called nosophobia
Hypengyophobia	responsibility		
Hypnophobia	falling asleep	Peniaphobia	poverty
Ichthyophobia	fish	Phagophobia	eating
Iophobia	poisons or rusty objects	Pharmacophobia	taking medicines
Keraunophobia	thunder and lightening	Phasmophobia	ghosts
Lalophobia	speaking or stuttering	Phobophobia	phobias
		Photophobia	light, or an abnormal sensitivity to light
Levophobia	objects to the left		
Molysmophobia	infection or contamination	Pnigophobia	choking
Mysophobia	dirt, being contaminated	Potamophobia	rivers or large bodies of water
Necrophobia	death or dead bodies	Pyrophobia	fire
		Scopophobia	being seen or stared at
Neophobia	novelty or the unknown	Taphephobia	being buried alive
Noctiphobia	night, with darkness and silence	Teratophobia	giving birth to a deformed baby
Nosophobia	disease		
Nyctophobia	darkness, night	Thalassophobia	the sea
Ochlophobia	crowds	Thanatophobia	death
Ombrophobia	rain	Theophobia	God
Ophidiophobia	snakes	Topophobia	being in a specific place
Panphobia	everything or an unknown evil	Toxicophobia	poisoning
		Triskaidekaphobia	the number 13
Paralipophobia	neglecting one's duty	Xenophobia	strangers
		Zelophobia	jealousy
Parasitophobia	parasites	Zoophobia	animals

Irrational Fears

A phobia is an intense, unrealistic fear of an object, an event, or a feeling. An estimated 18 percent of the U.S. adult population suffers from some kind of phobia, and a person can develop a phobia of anything—elevators, clocks, mushrooms, closed spaces, open spaces. Exposure to these trigger the rapid breathing, pounding heartbeat, and sweaty palms of panic.

There are three defined types of phobias:

- specific or simple phobias—fear of an object or situation, such as spiders, heights, or flying

- social phobias—fear of embarrassment or humiliation in social settings

- agoraphobia—fear of being away from a safe place.

No one knows for sure how phobias develop. Often, there is no explanation for the fear. In many cases, though, a person can readily identify an event or trauma—such as being chased by a dog—that triggered the phobia. What puzzles experts is why some people who experience such an event develop a phobia and others do not. Many psychologists believe the cause lies in a combination of genetic predisposition mixed with environmental and social causes.

Phobic disorders are classified as part of the group of anxiety disorders, which includes panic disorder, post-traumatic stress disorder, and obsessive-compulsive disorder. Several drugs regulated by the Food and Drug Administration are now being used to treat phobias and other anxiety disorders.

Dogs, Snakes, Dentists . . .

A person can develop a specific phobia of anything, but in most cases the phobia is shared by many and has a name. Animal phobias—cynophobia (dogs), equinophobia (horses), and zoophobia (all animals)—are common. So are arachnophobia (spiders) and ophidiophobia (snakes). And, of course, there's the fear of flying (pterygophobia), heights (acrophobia), and confined spaces (claustrophobia).

"One of the most common phobias is the fear of dentists," says Sheryl Jackson, Ph.D., a clinical psychologist and associate professor at the University of Alabama at Birmingham. "People who suffer with this phobia will literally let their teeth rot out because they are afraid to go to a dentist."

Jackson says that most specific phobias do not cause a serious disruption in a person's life, and, consequently, sufferers do not seek professional help. Instead, they find ways to avoid whatever it is that triggers their panic, or they simply endure the distress felt when they encounter it. Some may also consult their physicians, requesting medication to help them through a situation, such as an unavoidable plane trip for someone who is phobic about flying.

Drugs prescribed for these short-term situations include benzodiazepine antianxiety agents. These medications include two approved for treating anxiety disorders: Xanax (alprazolam) and Valium (diazepam). Beta blockers such as Inderal (propranolol) and Tenormin (atenolol), approved for controlling high blood pressure and some heart problems, have been acknowledged, partly on the basis of controlled trials, to be helpful in certain situations in which anxiety interferes with performance, such as public speaking.

Some phobias cause significant problems that require long-term professional help. "People usually seek treatment when their phobia interferes in their lives—the person who turns down promotions because he knows public speaking will be required, someone who must travel frequently but who is afraid of flying, or a woman who wants to have children but who has a fear of pain or blood. These are the people who seek long-term treatment," says Jackson.

While anti-anxiety medication sometimes may be used initially, systematic desensitization may also be an effective initial approach. Jackson explains that this non-drug treatment works on the theory that the more a person is exposed to the object of his phobia, the less fear that object generates.

First, the patient and therapist establish a hierarchy of feared situations, from the least to the most feared. For someone who fears elevators, for example, stepping onto the elevator causes a certain level of anxiety; going up one flight causes another level of anxiety. With each additional flight the anxiety increases until it becomes intolerable.

Therapy begins with the patient and therapist practicing the least fearful event, riding out the anxiety until the physiological symptoms subside. This step is repeated until the anxiety level is acceptable. Then the person progresses to the next step in the hierarchy. Each successive step is repeated until the physical reactions and anxious mood decrease to the point where the person can step onto an elevator and ride to the top floor without panicking.

✤ It's A Fact!!

Sometimes medications are used along with therapy in treating phobias. Some commonly used prescription medications include:

- Inderal (propranolol): helpful in certain situations in which anxiety interferes with performance

- Luvox (fluvoxamine) used for obsessive-compulsive disorder; sometimes used in treating social phobia

- Nardil (phenelzine): anti-anxiety drug sometimes used in treating social phobia

- Parnate (tranylcypromine): anti-anxiety drug sometimes used in treating social phobia

- Paxil (paroxetine): used for treatment of depression, obsessive-compulsive disorder, agoraphobia, panic disorder, and social phobia

- Prozac (fluoxetine): used for depression and obsessive-compulsive disorder; sometimes used in treating social phobia

- Tenormin (atenolol): helpful in certain situations in which anxiety interferes with performance

- Valium (diazepam): used for short-term, anxiety-producing situations

- Xanax (alprazolam): used for short-term, anxiety-producing situations

- Zoloft (sertraline): used for depression, obsessive-compulsive disorder; sometimes used in treating social phobia

Everyone's Looking At Me!

Social phobia is a complex disorder, characterized by the fear of being criticized or humiliated in social situations. There are two types of social phobias: circumscribed, which relates to a specific situation such as "stage fright," and generalized social phobia, which involves fear of a variety of social situations.

People suffering from social phobia fear the scrutiny of others. They tend to be highly sensitive to criticism, and often interpret the actions of others in social gatherings as an attempt to humiliate them. They are afraid to enter into conversations for fear of saying something foolish, and may agonize for hours or days later over things they did say.

"I always believed that everybody else knew the secret to enjoying themselves in social situations, that I was the only one who was so afraid," says Lorraine from Birmingham, Alabama, who asked that her last name not be used. "For a long time, I avoided as many situations as possible, even talking on the telephone. After a while, the loneliness and boredom would overwhelm me, and I would try again. I wanted to have fun, but I never really enjoyed myself because of the anxiety I felt. I always believed that others were looking at me and judging me."

Many people with social phobia are so sensitive to the scrutiny of others that they avoid eating or drinking in public, using public restrooms, or signing a check in the presence of another. Social phobia may often be associated with depression or alcohol abuse.

Neurotransmitter-receptor abnormalities in the brain are suspected to play a part in the development of social phobias. Neurotransmitters are substances such as norepinephrine, dopamine, and serotonin that are released in the brain. The substance then either excites or inhibits a target cell. Disorders in the physiology of these neurotransmitters are thought to be the cause of a variety of psychiatric illnesses.

Negative social experiences, such as being rejected by peers or suffering some type of embarrassment in public, and poor social skills also seem to be factors, and social phobia may be related to low self-esteem, lack of assertiveness, and feelings of inferiority.

Treatment can include cognitive-behavior therapy and medications, though no drug is approved specifically for social phobia. In addition to the anti-anxiety drugs and beta-blockers, medications may include the monoamine oxidase (MAO) inhibitor antidepressants Nardil (phenelzine) and Parnate (tranylcypromine), and serotonin specific reuptake inhibitors (SSRIs) such as Prozac (fluoxetine), Paxil (paroxetine), Zoloft (sertraline), and Luvox (fluvoxamine). Of the latter four drugs, Prozac, Zoloft and Paxil are approved for depression; Prozac, Paxil, Luvox, and Zoloft are approved for obsessive-compulsive disorder; and Paxil is approved for panic disorder.

Chris Sletten, Ph.D., a clinical psychologist and behavioral medicine specialist at the Mayo Clinic, says the use of SSRIs with behavior therapy is becoming more popular in the treatment of social phobia. Because there are fewer side effects associated with these drugs and a very low addiction potential, practitioners are more comfortable prescribing them. Plus, the antidepressant action of these drugs is helpful in treating patients who suffer from depression in addition to social phobia, he says.

✔ Quick Tip

Systematic desensitization may be an effective initial approach to the treatment of phobias. This non-drug treatment works on the theory that the more a person is exposed to the phobic object, the less fear that object generates. First, the patient and therapist establish a hierarchy of feared situations, from the least to the most feared. Therapy begins with the patient and therapist practicing the least fearful event, riding out the anxiety until the physiological symptoms subside. This step is repeated until the anxiety level is acceptable. Then the person progresses to the next step in the hierarchy. Each successive step is repeated until the physical reactions and anxious mood decrease to the point where the person can endure the feared situation without panicking.

"My therapist prescribed Prozac, and it has been an absolute godsend for me," Lorraine says. "After only a couple of months taking it, those voices in my head, the ones that always assured me that everyone was judging me—and finding me lacking—just seemed to shut up. I didn't feel high or drugged in any way. I felt like I always thought a "normal" person would feel. It's not a complete cure, of course. I still feel anxiety in social situations. But I don't avoid them as much. In fact, I actually pick up the phone now and ask friends to dinner, and I can relax enough to have fun. It's a whole new life for me."

The Wide Open Spaces

Agoraphobia comes from Greek, meaning literally "fear of the market-place," but it usually is defined as a fear of open spaces. Sletten says it stems more from the fear of being someplace where you will not be able to escape. It is closely identified with panic disorder, and in many cases, agoraphobia is directly related to the fear of experiencing a panic attack in public.

A person with panic disorder suffers sudden bouts of panic for no apparent reason. These attacks can occur anywhere at any time. One minute everything is fine, the next the person is engulfed by a feeling of terror. The heart races, breathing comes in gasps, and the entire body trembles. The attack may last only minutes, but its memory is etched indelibly in the brain, and the anticipation of another causes almost as much terror as the attack itself.

People who suffer agoraphobia avoid places and situations where they feel escape would be difficult in case an attack occurs. This could be anywhere—the grocery store, a shopping mall, the office. As the fear of an attack increases, the agoraphobic's world narrows to only a few places where he or she feels safe. In the most severe cases, this is limited to the home.

Agoraphobia is the most disabling of all the phobias, and treatment is difficult because there are so many associated fears—the fear of crowds, of elevators, of traffic. As with social phobias, treatment involves behavioral therapy combined with anti-anxiety or antidepressant medications, or both. Paxil has received FDA approval for use in treating panic disorders with or without agoraphobia, and at press time, Zoloft was being considered for this additional use.

"The most important thing for people with phobias to remember," says Sletten, "is that phobic disorders do respond well to treatment. It's not something they have to continue to suffer with."

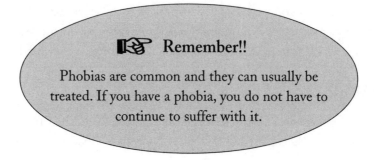

☞ Remember!!

Phobias are common and they can usually be treated. If you have a phobia, you do not have to continue to suffer with it.

Chapter 25

Social Phobia

Traumas And Treatments

When his self-described "worst episode" of anxiety lay hold of him on stage in 1994, Donny Osmond was no fledgling entertainer. The singer-actor had been in the public spotlight for more than 30 years—four of those, starting when he was just 18, as co-host of a popular variety program with his younger sister, Marie.

"Once the fear of embarrassing myself grabbed me," Osmond writes in his recent autobiography, *Life Is Just What You Make It*, "I couldn't get loose. It was as if a bizarre terrifying unreality had replaced everything that was familiar and safe. I felt powerless to think or reason my way out of the panic."

At the time, Osmond was playing the lead character in the Andrew Lloyd Webber musical "Joseph and the Amazing Technicolor Dreamcoat." "... I kept trying to remember the words," he continues, "but they slipped through my fingers like mercury, defying me to try again. The harder I tried, the more elusive they became. The best I could do was to not black out, and I got through the show, barely, by telling myself repeatedly, 'Stay conscious, stay conscious.'"

About This Chapter: Text in this chapter is from "Social Phobias," by Tamar Nordenberg in *FDA Consumer*, U.S. Food and Drug Administration, November 1999.

This was not garden-variety stage fright, Osmond explains. The entertainer who had confidently mixed with such stars as Bob Hope, John Wayne, Andy Griffith, Lucille Ball, Danny Thomas, and Farrah Fawcett, and who had won two celebrity auto races by driving his cars at speeds of up to 150 miles an hour, had become afraid—not just of humiliating himself during his shows, but of being scrutinized off-stage, as well, while doing things as mundane as returning merchandise to the store for a refund. The fear, Osmond says in his book, stemmed from the possibility of not always being in control of what happened to him. His mind would race: "What will I do? What will people think? Will I look stupid?"

As Osmond discovered, the condition that caused his foreboding panics had a name: social phobia. Also called social anxiety disorder, social phobia is an extreme fear of public embarrassment and being judged by others. The condition affects as many as 13 of every 100 Americans at some point in their lives, according to the Anxiety Disorders Association of America, making it the third most common psychiatric condition after substance abuse and depression.

> ✎ **Weird Words**
>
> Social Phobia: Fear and resulting avoidance of social situations in which a person would be noticed. One of the most common social phobias is the fear of public speaking.

To control his condition, Osmond learned techniques to manage his fears by changing his thought patterns. While many people address their social phobia with such psychological therapy alone, many others find medication helpful, either alone or coupled with psychotherapy. In May 1999, Paxil (paroxetine hydrochloride) became the first drug approved by the Food and Drug Administration specifically for treating social phobia.

Way Beyond Butterflies

Social phobia is far different from the run-of-the-mill nervousness associated with stressful situations. It's the intensity of the fear that distinguishes the condition from the almost inevitable butterflies that most people feel when they are about to give a speech or go to an interview or even a party.

When people with social phobia perceive that others will judge their "performance" in a certain situation, their bodies undergo physical changes, which typically include profuse sweating, rapid heartbeat, shortness of breath, faintness, and blushing.

"In the more severe cases, people can have a panic-like reaction and become so overwhelmed with anxiety that they feel completely disoriented," says Jerilyn Ross, president of the Anxiety Disorders Association of America and a psychotherapist who has treated thousands of patients with social phobia, including Osmond. "Your fight-or-flight alarm system that warns you when there's danger goes off at the wrong time. You literally feel like you're losing control, you're going to do something stupid to embarrass yourself, you're going to die."

Una McCann, M.D., an associate professor of psychiatry at the Johns Hopkins University School of Medicine and former head of the anxiety disorders unit at the National Institute of Mental Health, admits that when she started at NIMH, even she underestimated the life-altering impact that social phobia could have. "My initial reaction toward social phobia was probably typical of most people's," McCann says. "I thought, 'What's that? That's a disorder?' Because everybody experiences anxiety in some social situations, like public speaking, large crowds, or being the center of attention, it really seemed like a pseudo-disorder to me at first. Until I met some patients. Then, I suddenly realized how unbelievably debilitating social phobia can truly be."

For Marissa Turner, now 27 years old, even visiting her own aunt used to trigger panic-type symptoms. "It was pretty hair-raising," says Turner. "Standing on my aunt's doorstep, I'd be hyperventilating, shaking, and feeling hot when it wasn't hot outside. I'd feel like I wanted to turn around and run a mile. My throat would constrict, and it felt like if I opened my mouth to talk it wouldn't make a sound."

To avoid the frightening, panic-like reactions, people often rearrange their lives to sidestep their personal triggers rather than endure the intense anxiety. "What we're talking about is an anxiety so severe that a person is unable to function, either socially, academically, or occupationally," explains Thomas Laughren, M.D., the team leader for FDA's psychiatric drug products group. "You hear of people who would turn down a promotion or quit their job rather than dealing with talking to groups of people. Other people are shut-ins because they fear being judged in almost any social interaction outside of their family."

It's not that these people are shy, necessarily. Turner, for example, craved social interaction. "I could list a million things I wanted to do, which my peers were doing, that I couldn't," Turner says. "I didn't date. I rarely went to parties, and when I did, I was very scared the whole time."

Turner's condition is referred to as "generalized" social phobia because her anxiety extended to a broad variety of settings. Some people with generalized social phobia become very anxious about activities as routine as eating in a restaurant, writing something down while someone is watching, or using a public restroom. As a group, those with generalized social phobia are less likely to graduate from high school and are more likely to rely on government financial assistance or have poverty-level salaries, McCann points out.

Other people have the more limited "specific" social phobia, meaning their fear is associated with just public speaking or another well-defined circumstance.

Combination Of Causes

Scientists have not pinpointed the exact causes of social phobia, which tends to run in families and may affect women slightly more often than men. Studies suggest that both biological and psychological factors may contribute to the anxiety disorder.

Some scientists think social phobia is related to an imbalance of the brain chemical serotonin. Perhaps someone who is biologically predisposed to social phobia endures a triggering embarrassing event, Ross says. "I think we can all remember a time when we got up to talk, and the kids giggled because our skirt was up, or we forgot our line in a school play. At the moment it seemed like a traumatic experience, but for people who are biologically pre-disposed to social phobia, that experience can truly imprint itself on the brain as a traumatic event."

Many unproblematic years can pass between such an event and the phobia rearing its head, Ross says. Social phobia can appear any time in one's life, but typically shows up in the mid- to late-teens and can grow worse for a time after that, according to the Anxiety Disorders Association of America.

Turner has wrestled with her anxiety most of her life, but says that it "shot through the roof" as she neared adulthood. Like many fighting this war of nerves, Turner tried to self-medicate with alcohol. Without medical help, she says, she would have relied increasingly on drinking to get her through social situations. Turner did finally seek medical help, but not, she says, until she felt like she "couldn't cope with another day."

Addressing The Anxiety

Turner's doctor has prescribed the drug Paxil to ease the primary symp-toms of her social phobia. This first drug approved by FDA for treating the condition is also approved to treat depression, obsessive compulsive disorder, and an anxiety condition called panic disorder. However, it is not approved for performance anxiety or shyness that does not rise to the level of social phobia.

Paxil is an effective treatment option for doctors to consider, says the agency's Laughren, who adds that many patients will see improvement but not be cured of their anxiety altogether.

Turner says it has made a "really big difference" in her life. "Since I've started taking Paxil, I've been on top of my anxiety."

People taking antidepressant drugs called "monoamine oxidase inhibi-tors" shouldn't take Paxil. The drug should be used with particular caution in some other patients, such as those who are pregnant or nursing or who have a history of seizures, mania (emotional highs associated with bipolar disor-der), or certain other medical conditions.

✔ Quick Tip

Social Phobia Self-Test

If you suspect that you might suffer from social phobia, answer the following questions, and review your responses with your health care provider.

Yes or no? Are you troubled by:

• An intense and persistent fear of a social situation in which people might judge you?

• Fear that you will be humiliated by your actions?

• Fear that people will notice that you are blushing, sweating, trembling, or showing other signs of anxiety?

• Knowing that your fear is excessive or unreasonable?

Does the feared situation cause you to:

• Always feel anxiety?

• Experience a "panic attack," during which you suddenly are overcome by intense fear or discomfort, including any of these symptoms?

• pounding heart	• "jelly" legs
• sweating	• dizziness
• trembling or shaking	• feelings of unreality or being
• shortness of breath	detached from yourself
• fear of losing control, going crazy	• choking
	• fear of dying
• chest pain	• numbness or tingling sensations
• nausea or abdominal	• discomfort
• chills or hot flashes	

• Go to great lengths to avoid participating in the feared situation?

• Does all of this interfere with your daily life?

Having more than one illness at the same time can make it difficult to diagnose and treat the different conditions. Illnesses that sometimes complicate anxiety disorders include depression and substance abuse. With this in mind, please take a minute to answer the following questions:

- Have you experienced changes in sleeping or eating habits?

- More days than not, do you feel:

  - sad or depressed?

  - disinterested in life?

  - worthless or guilty?

- During the last year, has the use of alcohol or drugs:

  - Resulted in your failure to fulfill responsibilities with work, school, or family?

  - Placed you in a dangerous situation, such as driving a car under the influence?

  - Gotten you arrested?

  - Continued despite causing problems for you and/or your loved ones?

Reference

- *Diagnostic and Statistical Manual of Mental Disorders, Fourth Edition.* Washington, DC, American Psychiatric Association, 1994.

Source: Anxiety Disorders Association of America, 1190 Parklawn Drive, Suite 100, Rockville, MD 20852, USA. Reproduced with permission of the Anxiety Disorders Association of America.

Besides Paxil, doctors sometimes prescribe certain antidepressants or other drugs—beta blockers and benzodiazepines, for example—to try to control the anxiety symptoms associated with social phobia. While these drugs have not been approved by FDA specifically for treating social phobia, doctors can legally prescribe them if they feel a patient will benefit.

Some patients with social phobia opt for a non-drug treatment approach instead of, or in addition to, medication.

Philip Lawson (not his real name) is one of those who wanted to overcome his social anxiety without drugs. As an agent representing athletes, authors, and other public figures, the 24-year-old Lawson is required not only to meet individually with his clients and others, but also to give speeches. He relished doing presentations in college, but since graduating—during interviews and on his job as a talent representative—has battled an extreme fear of public speaking that's brought on white-knuckle anxiety attacks.

At first, Lawson didn't even want to accept that he had an anxiety disorder. "I'm the antithesis of someone you would expect to have a social problem. I planned my five-year high school reunion." The colleagues in whom he confided about his anxiety reacted with astonishment: "I don't believe it, you? Mister Outgoing Talk-to-Anybody?"

Yes, him, Lawson says. "When I had to give a presentation, I would either pretend to be unprepared or I'd say something really quick," he explains. "The anxiety grew into one-on-one meetings with people, where I would feel like I was completely on the spot. You always assume that all the attention is on you, like a spotlight."

Lawson's low point, he says, was when he called in sick to work because he had to give a speech. "I can either face this," he told himself, "or let it get worse and worse." Rather than allowing his condition to spiral downward, Lawson worked with a psychotherapist, individually and in group sessions, to learn to face down his irrational fears. He participated in a standard, two-pronged approach to treating social phobia called "cognitive-behavioral therapy."

The first part of cognitive-behavioral therapy—the "cognitive" aspect—tries to correct people's catastrophic perceptions of what others are thinking about them and what the real consequences are of a less-than-perfect performance. "Social phobia is a very self-focused illness," explains McCann. "You might think that people see you blushing and trembling, when really, many of them are thinking about what they're going to have for lunch."

To help people put things in perspective, a therapist may ask, "What is going to be the consequence if you do have a panic?" McCann's examples: "If you have a job interview and you blow it, so what? So you don't get that job. But it was good practice. So you do flub a sentence. What is the worst thing that can happen? Somebody might chuckle, maybe they'll rib you about it."

For Osmond, cognitive therapy reinforced what his wife, Debbie, had told him over and over: If he wasn't perfect, on-stage or off, people would like him nonetheless.

The "behavioral" aspect of therapy, typically undertaken at least partially in a group setting, gradually exposes people to the circumstances that can trigger their panic. It teaches them techniques to help them focus on the present reality rather than anticipating the imaginary dangers like "what if I lose control?" For example, people may learn to:

- expect the fear and accept rather than fight it.

- focus on manageable things in the present—by paying attention to their breathing, for example, or counting backwards from 100 by threes, repeating an encouraging phrase to themselves ("What doesn't kill me makes me stronger," for instance), picturing themselves at the beach or another place they would like to be, or consciously rubbing their hand on a podium, chair, or other object.

By socializing or giving a speech surrounded by an empathetic group, people can practice using these techniques to cope in the unnerving situation and give their confidence a boost. Speaking groups like Toastmasters might not be a sufficiently nurturing first step for those with social phobia, stresses Ross, who does encourage patients to join such groups once they conquer their paralyzing fear. "Toastmasters teaches you how to give an effective speech and deal with the normal fears and jitters," she says, "but it doesn't teach you how to deal with the more pathological anxiety."

Behavioral therapy homework assignments can include making presentations in a real-life environment. "It's not just going for those 12 or so weeks," McCann says. "You have to go through a little pain and have the failures to get your improvements."

Osmond's "homework" included a trip with Ross to the local shopping center to buy, and the next day return, a shirt. At the mall, he tracked his panics on a scale of 1 to 10 while practicing his coping tricks. "Now, the entire time I was in the mall," he writes, "my panic never went down to 0, but anything under 5 or so, I could cope with."

To this day, Lawson isn't entirely without anxiety, either, but says the quality of his life has improved significantly. "I went from calling in sick to now at least being able to get up in front of a group of people. I'm able to have one-on-one meetings with people without feeling terribly nervous. I try not to take myself so seriously."

Combined with her Paxil treatment, cognitive behavioral therapy contributed to Turner's progress, too. Paxil, she says, "calmed my nerves and elevated my mood enough that I could use all the cognitive behavioral therapy techniques I'd learned."

Taking Control

> **☞ Remember!!**
> Social phobia affects more than 13 percent of Americans. It is a real and serious health problem that responds to treatment. The first step is seeking help.

Up to 80 percent of those treated for social phobia say they've gotten their anxiety under control, according to the Anxiety Disorders Association of America. Yet a recent study reveals that treatment delays of 10 years or more are common among adults with the condition. Some reasons people cited for not being in treatment: a fear of what others might think, a belief that the anxiety could be controlled without professional help, and uncertainty about where to go.

But despite such hesitations, medical experts and individual sufferers alike urge people to seek out help for this real and treatable condition. Turner:

"The real me has been hidden for all these years. It's like a big, dark curtain was around me all that time, and I'm just now poking my head out. I want people to know they don't have to suffer. Life can be enjoyable."

As for Osmond, when his mind starts racing, he no longer thinks "what if I lose control?" Now, writes Osmond, he says to himself, "If I lose control, I know what to do."

Chapter 26

Post-Traumatic Stress Disorder

Post-traumatic stress disorder (PTSD) is an extremely debilitating condition that can occur after exposure to a terrifying event or ordeal in which grave physical harm was threatened or occurred. Traumatic events that can trigger PTSD include violent personal assaults such as rape or mugging, natural or man-made disasters, car accidents, or military combat.

♣ **It's A Fact!!**

Some studies have found the prevalence of post-traumatic stress disorder among adolescents to be as high as 8.1%. Other studies indicate that PTSD in teens increases the risk of alcohol and other drug abuse.

Most people with PTSD try to avoid any reminders or thoughts of the ordeal. Despite this avoidant behavior, many people with PTSD repeatedly re-experience the ordeal in the form of flashback episodes, memories, nightmares, or frightening thoughts, especially when they are exposed to events or objects reminiscent of the trauma. Symptoms of PTSD also include emotional numbness and sleep disturbances

About This Chapter: Text in this chapter is from an undated fact sheet on post-traumatic stress disorder produced by the National Institute of Mental Health.

(including insomnia), depression, and irritability or outbursts of anger. Feelings of intense guilt are also common. PTSD is diagnosed only if these symptoms last more than one month.

Fortunately, through research supported by the National Institute of Mental Health (NIMH), effective treatments have been developed to help people with PTSD.

> ✎ **Weird Words**
>
> Post-Traumatic Stress Disorder: A mental disorder with distinguishing symptoms following a traumatic event. The symptoms of post-traumatic stress disorder include re-experiencing the event, avoiding things associated with the event, dysfunctional thought processes, numbing of general responses, increased arousal, heightened startle reflex, insomnia, and nightmares.

How Common Is PTSD?

About 4% of the population will experience symptoms of PTSD in a given year.

When Does PTSD Strike?

PTSD can develop at any age, including childhood. Symptoms of PTSD typically begin within three months following a traumatic event, although occasionally symptoms do not begin until years later. Once PTSD develops, the duration of the illness varies. Some people recover within six months while others may suffer much longer.

What Treatments Are Available For PTSD?

Treatment for PTSD includes cognitive-behavioral therapy, group psychotherapy, and medications (including antidepressants). Various forms of exposure therapy (such as systemic desensitization and imaginal flooding) have all been used with PTSD patients. Exposure treatment for PTSD involves repeated reliving of the trauma, under controlled conditions, with the aim of facilitating the processing of the trauma.

Can People With PTSD Also Have Other Physical Or Emotional Illnesses?

People with PTSD can also have other psychological difficulties, particularly depression, substance abuse, or another anxiety disorder. The likelihood of treatment success is increased when these other conditions are appropriately diagnosed and treated, as well.

☞ **Remember!!**

Many adolescents at risk for developing post-traumatic stress disorder do not seek the help they need. Effective treatments are available, however. Treatment for PTSD includes cognitive-behavioral therapy, group psychotherapy, exposure therapy, and medications.

Chapter 27

Obsessive-Compulsive Disorder

What Is Obsessive-Compulsive Disorder (OCD)?

Obsessive-compulsive behavior is an anxiety disorder in which you are frequently or constantly troubled by ideas or images that stick in your mind and that you can't ignore (obsessions). These troubling and sometimes bizarre thoughts cause anxiety and compel you to behave in an unreasonable way. You may carry out repetitive, ritualistic acts (compulsions) to reduce this anxiety. Between 1% and 2.5% of the U.S. population suffers from OCD.

How Does It Occur?

The cause of obsessive-compulsive disorder (OCD) is unknown. The disorder may run in families. Men tend to begin experiencing the illness in their teenage years and women usually begin getting symptoms in their early 20s. Some studies have shown that the actual functioning of parts of the brain are different in people suffering from OCD. It used to be believed that OCD was caused by a deep unconscious conflict, but that theory is less supported today. The disorder is closely associated with mood disorders, including depression and bipolar disorder.

About This Chapter: Text in this chapter is from "Obsessive-Compulsive Disorder (OCD)," *Clinical Reference Systems*, July 1, 1999, p. 1082, © 1999 Clinical Reference Systems; reprinted with permission.

What Are The Symptoms?

People with OCD usually recognize that their obsessions or compulsions are preventing them from living fully and productively. They commonly describe their behavior as foolish or pointless, but they can't change it. Obsessional thoughts are often doubts about matters of safety (for example, shutting off the stove), but sometimes they have to do with a fear that something terrible will happen or that they will do something terrible, like kill loved ones for no reason. People with OCD may spend hours each day performing compulsive acts. The amount of time spent is less important than the degree of disruption caused in everyday life.

People with OCD often have depression or symptoms associated with depression. These include guilt, low self-esteem, anxiety, and extreme fatigue. However, many of these depressive symptoms can be secondary to the frustration brought on by an obsessive-compulsive problem. Obsessive-compulsive symptoms frequently create problems in interpersonal relationships and day-to-day functioning.

In extreme cases, people with OCD become totally disabled, have no friends, and can't leave home because they spend the day performing rituals or having obsessive thoughts.

✤ It's A Fact!!

Some of the typical compulsions or rituals of OCD are the following:

- **Cleaning:** Fearing germs, a person may shower repeatedly throughout the entire day or wash his or her hands until the skin is cracked and painful.

- **Repeating:** To reduce anxiety, a person may repeat a name or phrase many times.

- **Completing:** A person may perform a series of complicated steps in an exact order or repeat them until they are done perfectly.

- **Checking:** A person who fears harming himself or others by forgetting to lock the door or unplug the toaster will thus check repeatedly.

- **Hoarding:** A person may constantly collect useless items that he or she repeatedly counts and stacks.

How Is It Diagnosed?

There is no laboratory test for OCD. It is diagnosed by your doctor talking with you and someone close to you about your symptoms and asking very specific questions regarding the type of obsessions or compulsions you have. Your doctor may diagnose obsessive-compulsive disorder if your obsessions or compulsions cause you marked distress, take more than an hour of your time a day, or significantly interfere with your normal routine, occupation, social activities, or relationships with others.

Your doctor may ask you such questions as:

• Do you have troubling thoughts that you cannot ignore or get rid of regardless of how hard you try?

• Do you keep things extremely clean or wash your hands a lot, more so than other people you know?

• Do you check things over and over, even though you know that the oven has been turned off or that the front door is locked?

OCD is not concern about life's normal worries and your doctor will have to make sure that a medication or drug is not contributing to your symptoms. Also, phobias and chronic depression can occur along with OCD and it is important for your doctor to recognize which is which.

What Is The Treatment?

A combination of antidepressant drugs and behavior therapy has been most helpful in treating the disorder. Anafranil, Prozac, Zoloft, Paxil, and Luvox have been used with good results. In very rare circumstances neurosurgery is performed.

The type of behavior therapy most often used to treat OCD is called exposure and response prevention. It consists of having you confront your fears head-on by gradually exposing you to more and more of them and, while aided by your doctor, learning to suppress your obsessional thoughts and compulsive acts. If, for example, you wash your hands continually because you fear being dirty, your doctor may stand at the sink with you and prevent you from washing your hands until the anxiety goes away. This process also involves learning strategies for controlling your body's response to anxiety, such as breathing exercises.

How Long Will The Effects of Obsessive-Compulsive Disorder Last?

Obsessive-compulsive disorder usually appears in the late teens or early twenties. It may appear in childhood. Without treatment, the disorder may last a lifetime, becoming less severe from time to time, but rarely going away completely. In some people, OCD occurs in episodes, with years free of symptoms before a relapse. Developments in behavior therapy and new medications are helping many people with OCD live productive lives.

How Can I Take Care of Myself?

Include your family in your therapy. You and your family may benefit from reading books and viewing videotapes on OCD, and from attending support groups. Take your medication as recommended by your doctor and don't miss your behavioral therapy sessions.

✎ Weird Words

Compulsion: Uncontrollable impulses to perform a certain act for the purpose of alleviating fear or anxiety.

Obsession: A mental state characterized by a persistent, recurring, unwanted idea, often one that is recognized as senseless, but that cannot be eliminated.

Obsessive-Compulsive Disorder: A mental disorder marked by the persistent intrusion of unwanted ideas and the compulsion to perform repetitive, time-consuming acts (such as handwashing or touching) or ritualistic behaviors to relieve anxiety.

Know that you are not alone. There are millions of people affected by OCD and there are national organizations devoted to helping people with this disorder.

When Should I Call the Doctor?

Call your doctor if you feel that any of your ideas or actions are slipping out of your control.

Remember!!

Obsessive-compulsive behavior is a type of anxiety disorder affecting between 1% and 2.5% of the U.S. population.

For More Information

You can get more information about OCD from The Obsessive Compulsive Foundation, a worldwide, not-for-profit organization providing support and information to those who have OCD, their families and friends, and medical professionals. The address is:

The Obsessive Compulsive Foundation, Inc.
337 Notch Hill Road
North Branford, CT 06471
Phone: 203-315-2190
Fax: 203-315-2196
Website: http://www.ocfoundation.org
E-Mail: info@ocfoundation.org

Chapter 28

Computer Addiction

Computer addiction is real—an emerging disorder suffered by people who find that the virtual reality on computer screens is more attractive to them than everyday reality. This side effect of our changing technology may manifest itself at home, at school, and at work. Families, school counselors, and health care specialists have begun to notice the aberrant behavior and mental health problems of computer addicts.

As an impulse control disorder, computer addiction resembles pathological gambling. Addicts feel unhappy when they are away from the computer and try unsuccessfully to stop using it. They become preoccupied with thoughts about the computer and spend constantly increasing amounts of time and money on it, often neglecting their families and work. They then compound the problem by denying how much time and money they are spending. In one custody case involving a divorced couple, the husband claimed that his wife had neglected their children by spending 10 hours a day on the web. The court agreed that her use of the Internet was pathological and awarded custody to the father.

About This Chapter: Text in this chapter is from "Computer Addiction: Is It Real or Virtual?" excerpted from the January 1999 issue of the *Harvard Mental Health Letter*, © 1999, by the President and Fellow of Harvard College; reprinted with permission. This article is based on an interview with Maressa Hecht Orzack, Ph.D., Founder and Coordinator, Computer Addiction Services, McLean Hospital, and Lecturer in Psychology in the Department of Psychiatry at Harvard Medical School.

Anyone who uses a computer is vulnerable, but especially people who are easily bored, lonely, shy, depressed, or suffering from other addictions.

They may rely on the computer screen to solve personal problems or meet their needs for companionship, belonging, or even sexual fulfillment. The many links in the World Wide Web offer endless new connections in a progression that draws addicts in ever further. Like gambling, computer addiction provides a reinforcement pattern known as variable ratio schedule—rewards come more or less at random rather than in a fixed arrangement.

Animal experiments show that behavior resulting in this pattern is the slowest to be extinguished (eliminated) when the rewards are withdrawn. A man who had a romantic encounter with what he thought was his perfect fantasy match was horrified to discover that his virtual companion was not the person he imagined, but soon afterward he became excited again by another "perfect match."

✎ **Weird Words**

Impulse-Control Disorder: A mental disorder in which a person fails to resist an urge to do something harmful to him/herself or others. Kleptomania (impulsive stealing), trichotillomania (hair pulling), and pathologic gambling are all examples of impulse-control disorders.

The two main options for treatment are cognitive-behavioral therapy (CBT) and motivational enhancement therapy (MET). CBT is a familiar treatment based on the premise that thoughts determine feelings. Patients are taught to monitor their thoughts and identify those that trigger addictive feelings and actions while they learn new coping skills and ways to prevent a relapse. CBT usually requires three months of weekly therapeutic sessions along with telephone checkups.

MET is less familiar. Its aim is to help patients acknowledge that they have a problem and need to change their behavior. The stages of change are contemplation, determination, action, maintenance, and contemplation again after a relapse. The therapy requires four sessions in three months, and the methods are summarized by the acronym FRAMES: feedback, responsibility, advice, menu, empathy, self-efficiency.

- **Feedback:** The therapist assesses the computer use of patients in great detail and reaffirms their acknowledgment of the need for help.

- **Responsibility:** Patients are told that they are responsible for changing their behavior.

- **Advice:** Patient and therapist together work out the goals, which include learning how to recognize the difference between healthy and addictive computer use.

- **Menu:** A schedule is devised by which the patient monitors computer use and the associated thoughts and feelings.

- **Empathy:** The efforts of patients are constantly reaffirmed, and they are not scolded for slips or failures.

- **Self-efficiency:** Patients learn to use the computer mainly for work, with the help of feedback through telephone contacts with the therapist. In the last session, therapist and patient review progress, renew motivation, and reaffirm the patient's commitment to change.

☞ **Remember!!**

Anyone who uses a computer is at risk for developing computer addiction, but people who are easily bored, lonely, shy, depressed, or suffering from other addictions are especially vulnerable.

Chapter 29

Personality Disorders

The character of a person is shown through his or her personality—by the way an individual thinks, feels, and behaves. When the behavior is inflexible, maladaptive, and antisocial, then that individual is diagnosed with a personality disorder.

Most personality disorders begin as problems in personal development and character which peak during adolescence and then are defined as personality disorders.

Personality disorders are not illnesses in a strict sense as they do not disrupt emotional, intellectual, or perceptual functioning. However, those with personality disorders suffer a life that is not positive, proactive, or fulfilling. Not surprisingly, personality disorders are also associated with failures to reach potential.

The *DSM-IV: Diagnostic and Statistical Manual of Mental Disorders* (American Psychiatric Association) defines a personality disorder as an enduring pattern of inner experience and behavior that deviates markedly from the expectation of the individual's culture, is pervasive and inflexible, has an onset in adolescence or early adulthood, is stable over time, and leads to distress or impairment.

About This Chapter: Text in this chapter was written by Linda Lebelle, Director of Focus Adolescent Services, Salisbury, MD. © 2000 Focus Adolescent Services; reprinted with permission. For more information on teens' mental health concerns, visit Focus Adolescent Services' website at http://www.focusas.com or call toll free 1-877-362-8727.

Identifying The Disorders

Currently, there are 10 distinct personality disorders identified in the *DSM-IV*:

- **Antisocial Personality Disorder:** Lack of regard for the moral or legal standards in the local culture, marked inability to get along with others or abide by societal rules. Sometimes called psychopaths or sociopaths.

- **Avoidant Personality Disorder:** Marked social inhibition, feelings of inadequacy, and extremely sensitive to criticism.

✎ Weird Words

<u>Affect:</u> Pertaining to mood or emotion.

<u>Delusion Of Grandeur:</u> An exaggerated belief in one's own importance, wealth, or power.

<u>*Diagnostic and Statistical Manual IV (DSM-IV)*</u>: Complete title of this book, which is produced by the American Psychiatric Association, is *Diagnostic and Statistical Manual of Mental Disorders, Fourth Edition*. It provides standard names and descriptions of mental disorders; these terms and guidelines are used by health care providers in making diagnostic assessments. The first edition was published in 1952; the fourth edition, which is the most recent, was published in 1994.

<u>Emotion:</u> A strong feeling such as joy, anger, or fear, accompanied by psychological changes and arising without conscious effort; often demonstrated with alterations in behavior.

<u>Empathy:</u> To be able to understand and communicate the understanding of someone else's emotions and feelings.

<u>Obsession:</u> A mental state characterized by a persistent, recurring, unwanted idea, often one that is recognized as senseless, but that cannot be eliminated.

- **Borderline Personality Disorder:** Lack of one's own identity, with rapid changes in mood, intense unstable interpersonal relationships, marked impulsively, instability in affect and in self image.

- **Dependent Personality Disorder:** Extreme need of other people, to a point where the person is unable to make any decisions or take an independent stand on his or her own. Fear of separation and submissive behavior. Marked lack of decisiveness and self-confidence.

♣ **It's A Fact!!**

Most personality disorders begin as problems in personal development and character which peak during adolescence.

- **Histrionic Personality Disorder:** Exaggerated and often inappropriate displays of emotional reactions, approaching theatricality, in everyday behavior. Sudden and rapidly shifting emotion expressions.

- **Narcissistic Personality Disorder:** Behavior or a fantasy of grandiosity, a lack of empathy, a need to be admired by others, an inability to see the viewpoints of others, and hypersensitive to the opinions of others.

- **Obsessive-Compulsive Personality Disorder:** Characterized by perfectionism and inflexibility; preoccupation with uncontrollable patterns of thought and action.

- **Paranoid Personality Disorder:** Marked distrust of others, including the belief, without reason, that others are exploiting, harming, or trying to deceive him or her; lack of trust; belief of others' betrayal; belief in hidden meanings; unforgiving and grudge holding.

- **Schizoid Personality Disorder:** Primarily characterized by a very limited range of emotion, both in expression of and experiencing; indifferent to social relationships.

- **Schizotypal Personality Disorder:** Peculiarities of thinking, odd beliefs, and eccentricities of appearance, behavior, interpersonal style, and thought (for example, belief in psychic phenomena and having magical powers).

Common Elements In Personality Disorders

According to Dr. Sam Vaknin, author of *Malignant Self-Love: Narcissism Revisited*, individuals with personality disorders have many things in common.

- Self-centeredness that manifests itself through a me-first, self-preoccupied attitude.

- Lack of individual accountability that results in a victim mentality and blaming others, society and the universe for their problems.

- Lack of perspective-taking and empathy.

- Manipulative and exploitative behavior.

- Unhappiness, suffering from depression and other mood and anxiety disorders.

- Vulnerability to other mental disorders, such as obsessive-compulsive tendencies and panic attacks.

- Distorted or superficial understanding of self and others' perceptions, being unable to see his or her objectionable, unacceptable, disagreeable, or self-destructive behaviors or the issues that may have contributed to the personality disorder.

- Socially maladaptive, changing the rules of the game, introducing new variables, or otherwise influencing the external world to conform to their own needs.

- No hallucinations, delusions, or thought disorders (except for the brief psychotic episodes of Borderline Personality Disorder).

Vaknin does not propose a unified theory of psychopathology as there is still much to learn about the workings of the world and our place in it. Each personality disorder shows its own unique manifestations through a story or narrative, but we do not have enough information or verifying capability to determine whether they spring from a common psychodynamic source.

It is important to note that some people diagnosed with borderline, antisocial, schizoid, and obsessive-compulsive personality disorders may be suffering from an underlying biological disturbance (anatomical, electrical, or neurochemical). A strong genetic link has been found in antisocial and borderline personality disorders.

Treatment Of Personality Disorders

By reading the *DSM-IV*'s definition of personality disorders, it may seem that these conditions are not treatable. However, when individuals choose to be in control of their lives and are committed to changing their lives, healing is possible. Therapy and medications can help, but it is the individual's decision to take accountability for his or her own life that makes the difference.

To heal, individuals must first have the desire to change in order to break through the enduring pattern of a personality disorder. Individuals need to want to gain insight into and face their inner experience and behavior. (These issues may concern severe or repeated trauma during childhood, such as abuse.)

This involves changing their thinking—about themselves, their relationships, and the world. This also involves changing their behavior, for that which is not acted upon is not learned.

Then, with a support system (for example, therapy, self-help groups, friends, family, medication), they can free themselves from their imprisoned life.

☞ Remember!!

A personality disorder is identified by a pervasive pattern of experience and behavior that is abnormal with respect to any of the following two: thinking, mood, personal relations, and the control of impulses. To heal, individuals must first have the desire to change.

Chapter 30

Attention Deficit Disorder

Pete's Story

Pete is thoughtfully answering a question about how he's adjusted to life as a college freshman and what it's like to manage his daily routine entirely on his own. Abruptly, in the middle of a sentence, he hesitates.

"Excuse me," he says after a moment's silence, "but could you please repeat the question?"

Pete is good-looking—tall, blonde, and athletic—and extremely good-natured. Even now, when you think he might be embarrassed by his lapse, he reacts with a broad smile.

It isn't unusual for his mind to wander off a subject. This happens, in fact, all the time. Pete has attention deficit disorder (ADD), the most common psychiatric disorder among young people, affecting an estimated 3 percent to 5 percent of all school-age children—mainly boys. At least two-thirds of these young people carry this disability into adulthood.

People who have the disorder consistently show certain characteristic behaviors over a period of time. The most common behaviors fall into three categories: inability to pay attention, hyperactivity, and impulsivity.

About This Chapter: Text in this chapter is from "Pete's Story," by Nancy Dreher, in *Current Health 2*, September 1998, © 1998 Weekly Reader Corporation; reprinted with permission.

Like many other teens with ADD, Pete succeeds in spite of his condition—some would say because of it. He's doing well as a college freshman. At his Illinois high school, he was an active student and athlete. He also used many forums to explain ADD to others—including an informational video he made as part of the project that earned him his rank as an Eagle Scout.

Dealing With ADD

Pete's story is positive for many reasons. For one thing, he knows exactly what his particular disabilities are and understands them. For another, he's learned how to carefully organize his school assignments and other daily activities. He takes medicine that works and he has a lot of support from his family.

These factors can be the cornerstone of dealing with ADD as a teen, when responsibilities increase, schoolwork is more demanding, and social life usually assumes a higher priority.

Most teens with ADD have lived with their diagnosis for several years, since about 70 percent of young people with ADD get diagnosed before middle school. Regardless of when the diagnosis is made, however, learning to adapt to ADD is a challenge.

Meeting the challenge is important because so many young people with ADD continue to have their disability as adults. This does not limit their potential. In fact, many adults with ADD become very resourceful, even using certain attributes of ADD to help them excel in their careers. They are able to focus on their strengths and develop strategies that work for them.

> ✎ **Weird Words**
>
> Attention-Deficit Hyperactivity Disorder (ADHD): A behavioral disorder characterized by a pattern of inattention, excessive activity, learning disabilities, and disruptive behavior which is usually observed in family, school, and social settings.
>
> Hyperactivity: Excessive movement and general restlessness. Behaviors frequently seen in children who are considered hyperactive include impulsivity, distractibility, difficulty concentrating, and aggressiveness.

What Exactly Is ADD?

ADD is clinically known as attention deficit hyperactivity disorder (ADHD). The term ADHD covers three patterns of extreme behavior. People with ADHD may show several signs of being unable to pay attention. They may have a pattern of being hyperactive or impulsive. Or, they may show all three types of behavior.

Everyone shows some of these behaviors at times, but in people with ADHD these behaviors occur often and in extremes, have been happening for a long time, and affect more than one area of their life.

Symptoms Of Inattention:

- Fails to pay close attention to details or makes careless mistakes in schoolwork, work, or other activities
- Has difficulty sustaining attention in tasks or play activities
- Does not seem to listen when spoken to directly
- Does not follow through on instructions and fails to finish schoolwork, chores, or duties in the workplace
- Has difficulty organizing tasks and activities
- Avoids, dislikes, or is reluctant to engage in tasks that require sustained mental effort
- Loses things necessary for tasks or activities
- Easily distracted by irrelevant sights and sounds
- Forgetful in daily activities

Symptoms Of Hyperactivity:

- Fidgets with hands or feet or squirms in a seat
- Leaves a seat early in a classroom or in other situations
- Runs about or climbs excessively at inappropriate times
- Has difficulty playing or engaging in leisure activities quietly

- Is often "on the go" or acts as if "driven by a motor"
- Talks excessively
- Blurts out answers before questions have been completed
- Has difficulty awaiting a turn
- Interrupts or intrudes on others

ADD is believed to be caused by a lower level of activity in the parts of the brain that inhibit impulses and control attention. There is a great deal of evidence that ADD runs in families. According to the National Attention Deficit Disorder Association, recent studies show that if one person in a family is diagnosed with ADD, there is a strong probability that another family member could also have ADD.

*Source: *Diagnostic and Statistical Manual of the American Psychiatric Association (Revision IV).*

How Medication Can Help

When a diagnosis of ADD is made—regardless of the patient's age—one of the first steps a physician considers is whether to prescribe drugs as treatment. Medications in the class of drugs known as stimulants seem to be the most effective in treating both children and adults with ADD. These include methylphenidate (Ritalin) and dextroamphetamine (Dexedrine, Adderall, and generics). Some antidepressants are also prescribed for ADD. For many people with ADD, medication dramatically reduces hyperactivity and improves the ability to focus, work, and learn. The medications also may improve physical coordination, such as handwriting, and success in sports.

Many young people with ADD don't like the idea of taking daily doses of medicine, regardless of whether it helps them. Experts point out, however, that taking ADD medication is comparable to wearing glasses or braces or taking allergy medication—something that no one regards as abnormal or unusual. It's important to remember, too, that when there are improvements in schoolwork or behavior, it's not the drug itself that is responsible. Credit for that goes to the student, who has simply been helped by the drug to perform to the best of his or her ability.

Stimulant Medicine: Potential For Abuse?

A lot of attention has been paid in recent years to the potential for abuse of stimulants used in ADD treatment, but medical professionals point out that if prescribed and taken properly, these drugs are not addictive.

Nor does the use of stimulants by children lead to drug addiction later in life. By enabling young people to focus and be more successful, medication can help them avoid negative experiences and actually help prevent addictions and other emotional problems later.

The U.S. Drug Enforcement Administration has placed strict controls on the manufacture, distribution, and prescription of stimulant medicines. Drug manufacturers have also made an effort to make physicians and patients aware of the risks of abuse.

People who take ADD medication have the responsibility to know the name, dose, and timing of their medicine—and not to share it with anyone else.

> ♣ **It's A Fact!!**
>
> Attention deficit disorder (ADD) affects an estimated 3 to 5 percent of school-age children. The majority of ADD patients are boys.

Skills And Willpower

On the other hand, some people think that drugs can solve any problem created by ADD, or even cure the disorder. Neither is true. Medication can help, but for teens especially, one of the best treatments involves learning skills that make it possible for them to help themselves. These skills revolve around organization and structure, both at home and school.

Pete, for example, lives by his "plan," a master schedule that he writes down by hand (and also keeps on a computer). He breaks down his daily schedule into segments. There is a specific amount of time set aside for studying each subject, for meals, and for free time.

He's found that it also helps to talk about what he needs to do, to put his "plan" in words and to describe it to his mom at home and a teacher at school.

In high school, he learned that speaking his ideas out loud sometimes helped him focus more clearly on his work. After arranging to take some exams orally, for example, he saw his grades improve.

Then there's his computer. His fingers can fly over the keyboard and keep up with his thoughts at a speed that was never possible with longhand. When writing things out by hand, he was distracted by the effort he was putting into his penmanship.

Having a secret weapon helps, too. When he's asked how he so effectively deals with ADD, the first concept he mentions is willpower. He says he uses willpower to force himself to concentrate, to keep his head and his hands still, and to stick to the "plan." But fortunately, his willpower can't do anything to stop his smile.

☞ Remember!!

Attention deficit disorder is the most common psychiatric disorder among young people. Teens with ADD generally must be treated by a professional or a team of professionals in order to experience long-term improvement. Learning to adapt to ADD is a challenge. Learning to cope with ADD is a challenge, but it does not limit a teen's potential.

For more information visit the National Attention Deficit Disorder Association's website at:

http://www.add.org

Chapter 31

Eating Disorders

Eating disorders are real and serious illnesses that can sometimes be life-threatening. They are also very common. Each year, more than five million Americans have an eating disorder. Most of these individuals are teens and young adult women, but eating disorders are also common among gay men, victims of sexual abuse, and male athletes who are involved in sports with weight classes.

The major types of eating disorders are anorexia nervosa, bulimia, and binge eating disorder. Approximately one percent of teenage girls develop anorexia nervosa. Another two to three percent of young women develop bulimia nervosa. Binge eating disorder is found in about two percent of the general population—more often in women than men. Recent research shows that binge eating disorder occurs in about 30 percent of people participating in medically supervised weight control programs.

It is very likely that you know someone who has an eating disorder. The good news is that there is hope. Learning how to identify these disorders can help you to help yourself or a friend with an eating disorder. With treatment, people do get better and can return to their everyday lives.

About This Chapter: Text in this chapter is from "Teen Eating Disorders," a pamphlet produced by the National Mental Health Association (NMHA), © 1997, revised February 2001. Reprinted with permission from the National Mental Health Association (1-800-969-NMHA).

Anorexia Nervosa

People who intentionally starve themselves have an eating disorder called anorexia nervosa. The disorder, which usually begins in young people around the time of puberty and involves extreme weight loss—at least 15 percent below the individual's normal body weight. Many people with the disorder look extremely thin but are convinced they are overweight. For reasons not yet understood, they become terrified of gaining any weight. Sometimes they must be hospitalized to prevent starvation. One in ten cases of anorexia nervosa leads to death from starvation, cardiac arrest, other medical complications or suicide.

Medical complications of anorexia include:

- starvation which can damage vital organs such as the heart and brain
- monthly menstrual periods stop
- breathing, pulse, and blood pressure rates drop, and thyroid function slows
- nails and hair become brittle
- the skin dries, yellows, and becomes covered with soft fine hair
- excessive thirst and frequent urination may occur
- mild anemia, swollen joints, reduced muscle mass
- bones may become brittle and prone to breakage.

> ♣ **It's A Fact!!**
>
> Warning signs for *anorexia nervosa*:
>
> A person may ...
>
> - not eat enough
> - feel "fat" even if he or she is very thin
> - always feel cold and tired
> - exercise vigorously at odd hours

Bulimia Nervosa

People with bulimia nervosa consume large amounts of food and then rid their bodies of the excess calories by vomiting, abusing laxatives or diuretics, taking enema

Some use a combination of all these forms of purging. Because many individuals with bulimia "binge and purge" in secret and maintain normal or above normal body weight, they can often successfully hide their problem from others for years.

Medical complications of bulimia nervosa include:

- an irregular heartbeat

- dehydration (the body doesn't have enough water)

- tooth decay from the stomach acid found in vomit

- cuts and scrapes on the backs of hands when fingers are pushed down the throat to induce vomiting.

❖ **It's A Fact!!**

Warning signs for *bulimia nervosa*:

A person may ...

- Eat a lot of food quickly, then get rid of it by purging vomiting or misusing laxatives or diuretics (drugs that increase urination)

- gain and lose weight often

- have irregular menstrual periods

- starve himself or herself after eating instead of purging

Binge Eating Disorder

An illness that resembles bulimia nervosa is binge eating disorder. Like bulimia, this disorder is characterized by episodes of uncontrolled eating or bingeing. However, binge eating disorder differs from bulimia because its sufferers do not purge their bodies of excess food. In contrast to other eating disorders, one-third to one-fourth of all patients with binge eating disorders are men.

Medical complications of binge eating disorder include:

- serious medical problems associated with obesity, such as high cholesterol, high blood pressure, and diabetes.

❖ **It's A Fact!!**

Warning signs for *binge eating disorder*: A person may ...

- not stop eating when full

- become obese or gain weight rapidly

- eat a lot of food in a short time without purging afterwards

Why Do Teens Develop Eating Disorders?

There may be more than one reason a person develops an eating disorder.

- **A person's self image:** Most teens with eating disorders share certain personality traits: low self-esteem, feelings of helplessness, and a fear of becoming fat.

- **The need to be perfect:** People with anorexia tend to be "too good to be true." They rarely disobey, keep their feelings to themselves, and tend to be perfectionists, good students and excellent athletes. Having followed the wishes of others for the most part, they have not learned how to cope with the problems typical of adolescence, growing up, and becoming independent.

- **A stressful personal life:** People who develop bulimia and binge eating disorder typically consume huge amounts of food—often junk food— to reduce stress and relieve anxiety. With binge eating, however, come

✎ **Weird Words**

Anorexia Nervosa: An eating disorder characterized by an aversion to eating, excessive fasting, extreme and sometimes life-threatening weight loss, and fear of being fat. Anorexia nervosa is most often diagnosed in adolescent girls, and it is frequently accompanied by a distorted body image, feelings of being fat even if the patient is very thin, excessive activity, and amenorrhea (absence of menstruation).

Binge Eating Disorder: An eating disorder characterized by secretive episodes of uncontrolled eating in which large amounts of food are eaten in a short time. Unlike builima nervosa, the eating episodes are not followed by self-induced vomiting or other means of purging.

Bulimia Nervosa: An eating disorder characterized by repeated, secretive episodes of binge eating followed by self-induced vomiting, laxative abuse, or excessive exercise to avoid gaining weight. Periods of bulimic behavior can alternate with periods of normal eating or fasting.

guilt and depression. Purging can bring relief, but it is only temporary. Individuals with bulimia are also impulsive and more likely to engage in risky behavior such as abuse of alcohol and drugs.

- **Genetics** (traits a person inherits from parents): Eating disorders appear to run in families—with female relatives most often affected.

- **Society or family pressures:** Girls with eating disorders often have fathers, mothers, and/or brothers who are overly critical of their weight. People pursuing professions or activities that emphasize thinness—like modeling, dancing, gymnastics, wrestling, and long-distance running—are more susceptible to the problem.

♣ It's A Fact!!

Many teens with eating disorders also have other mental illnesses such as clinical depression, anxiety, post-traumatic stress disorder, personality or substance abuse disorders, and many are at risk for suicide. Obsessive-compulsive disorder (OCD), an illness characterized by repetitive thoughts and behavior, can also accompany anorexia or bulimia. Individuals with anorexia are eager to please, but may have sudden outbursts of hostility and anger, or become socially withdrawn. Research his shown that individuals with binge eating disorder have high rates of co-occurring mental disorders—especially depression.

- **The body's chemistry:** In the central nervous system—particularly the brain—key chemical messengers known as neurotransmitters control hormone production. Recently, scientists have learned that these neurotransmitters are decreased in acutely ill people with anorexia and bulimia and long-term recovered anorexia patients.

Treatment

Eating disorders are most successfully treated when diagnosed early. The first step is a complete physical examination to rule out any other illnesses.

Once an eating disorder is diagnosed, a doctor must determine whether the person is in immediate medical danger and requires hospitalization.

Treatment plans usually include a combination of:

- **Cognitive behavioral therapy:** Learning new patterns of behavior with food and relationships.

- **Psychotherapy:** Talking out problems with a trained professional and finding ways to solve them. Individual, group, and family therapy are often recommended.

- **Nutrition counseling:** Understanding proper nutrition, restoring normal body weight, and learning to eat in a healthy manner are critical to recovery.

- **Medication:** Certain drugs may be prescribed to relieve depression, anxiety, and bingeing. Studies show that antidepressants can be used successfully to treat some people with eating disorders.

While most people can be treated in an outpatient setting, some may need hospital care. Hospitalization may be necessary if a person experiences:

- excessive and rapid weight loss
- severe binge eating and purging
- serious medical complications
- clinical depression and suicidal thoughts

☞ Remember!!

Eating disorders are common illnesses that can sometimes be life-threatening. They are most successfully treated when diagnosed early. For more information or referrals for local services, contact your local mental health association or the National Mental Health Association (Toll-Free: 800-969-6642). You may also want to check these sources on the Internet:

Academy for Eating Disorders
http://www.acadeatdis.org

Anorexia Nervosa and Related Eating Disorders, Inc. (ANRED)
http://www.anred.com

National Eating Disorders Association
http://www.edap.org

National Eating Disorders Organization
http://www.kidsource.com/nedo

National Mental Health Association
http://www.nmha.org

Chapter 32

Body Dysmorphic Disorder

What Is Body Dysmorphic Disorder?

People with body dysmorphic disorder (BDD) worry about some aspect of their appearance. They worry, for example, that their skin is scarred, their hair is thinning, their nose is too big, or something else is wrong with how they look. When others tell them that they look fine or that the flaw they perceive is minimal, people with this disorder find it hard to believe this reassurance.

People with BDD think a lot about their perceived appearance flaw, generally for at least an hour a day. Some say they're obsessed. Most find that they don't have as much control over their thoughts about the body flaw as they would like.

In addition, the appearance concern causes significant distress (for example, anxiety or depression) or it causes significant problems in functioning. Although some people with this disorder manage to function well despite their distress, many find that their appearance concerns cause problems for them. For example, they may find it hard to concentrate on their job or school work, which may suffer, and relationship problems are common. People with

About This Chapter: Text in this chapter is excerpted from "Body Dysmorphic Disorder (BDD) and Body Image Program," prepared by Butler Hospital, Providence, Rhode Island and posted at http://www.butler.org/bdd.html, © Butler Hospital; reprinted with permission.

BDD may have few friends, avoid dating, miss school, and feel very self-conscious in social situations.

The severity of BDD varies. Some people experience manageable distress and are able to function well, although not up to their potential. Others find that this disorder ruins their life.

✎ **Weird Words**

Dysmorphic: Abnormally shaped. Body dysmorphic disorder is a mental disorder in which a person is preoccupied with imagined bodily faults.

Obsession: A mental state characterized by a persistent, recurring, unwanted idea, often one that is recognized as senseless, but that cannot be eliminated.

How Do I Know If I Really Have BDD?

You can ask yourself the following set of questions to determine whether you might have BDD.

1. Are you very concerned about the appearance of some parts(s) of your body which you consider especially unattractive?

   If yes: Do these concerns preoccupy you? That is, you think about them a lot and wish you could worry less?

2. How much time do you spend thinking about your defect(s) per day on average? (add up all the time you spend)

   a. Less than 1 hour a day

   b. 1-3 hours a day

   c. More than 3 hours a day

3. Is your main concern with your appearance that you aren't thin enough or that you might become too fat?

4. What effect has your preoccupation with your appearance had on your life?

> Has your defect(s) often caused you a lot of distress, torment, or pain?

> Has your defect(s) often significantly interfered with your social life?

> Has your defect(s) often significantly interfered with your school work, your job, or your ability to function in your role (e.g., as a homemaker)?

> Are there things you avoid because of your defect(s)?

You're likely to have BDD if you gave the following answers:

1. Yes to both parts.

2. Answer B or C.

3. While a "yes" answer may indicate that BDD is present, it is possible that an eating disorder is a more accurate diagnosis.

4. Yes to any of the questions.

Please note that the above questions are intended to screen for BDD, not diagnose it; the answers indicated above can suggest that BDD is present but can't necessarily give a definitive diagnosis.

Clues To The Presence Of BDD

The questions listed above ask about the features of BDD that are required for the diagnosis. BDD also has some features that, while not necessary for the diagnosis, can provide clues to its presence, some of which are the following:

1. Frequently comparing your appearance with that of others; scrutinizing the appearance of others.

2. Often checking your appearance in mirrors and other reflecting surfaces.

3. Camouflaging the perceived defect with clothing, makeup, a hat, your hand, your posture, or in some other way.

4. Seeking surgery, dermatological treatment, or other medical treatment for appearance concerns when doctors or other people have said your flaws are minimal or such treatment isn't necessary.

5. Questioning: seeking reassurance about the flaw or attempting to convince others of its ugliness.

6. Excessive grooming (for example, combing hair, shaving, removing or cutting hair, applying makeup)

7. Avoiding mirrors.

8. Frequently touching the perceived defect.

9. Picking your skin.

10. Measuring the disliked body part.

11. Excessively reading about the defective body part.

12. Exercising or dieting excessively.

13. Using drugs (for example, anabolic steroids) to become more muscular or lose fat.

> ✤ **It's A Fact!!**
> BDD is often misdiagnosed as another psychiatric disorder. This occurs because BDD can produce symptoms that mimic other disorders such as social phobia, agoraphobia, panic disorder, trichotillomania (hair pulling), obsessive compulsive disorder, and depression.

14. Avoiding social situations in which the perceived defect might be exposed.

15. Feeling very anxious and self-conscious around other people because of the perceived defect.

BDD Is Often Underdiagnosed

The diagnosis of BDD is often missed because of:

-   **Secrecy and shame:** Many people with BDD don't reveal their symptoms to others because of embarrassment.

- **Lack of familiarity with BDD:** Many, including health professionals, are not aware that BDD is a known psychiatric disorder that often responds to psychiatric treatment.

- **Trivialization:** BDD is easily trivialized, even though it is a serious and distressing condition.

- **Pursuit of non-psychiatric, medical, and surgical treatment:** Many people with BDD see dermatologists, plastic surgeons, and other physicians rather than mental health professionals. These treatments often are not helpful.

Hope For BDD Sufferers

There is hope for BDD sufferers. Psychiatric treatment is often effective in decreasing BDD symptoms and the suffering it causes. The treatments that appear most effective are certain psychiatric medications and a type of therapy known as cognitive-behavioral therapy.

The medications that are most promising are serotonin reuptake inhibitors (SRIs). These medications are fluvoxamine (Luvox), fluoxetine (Prozac), sertraline (Zoloft), paroxetine (Paxil), citalopram (Celexa) and clomipramine (Anafranil). These medications are not addicting and are usually well tolerated. They can significantly relieve BDD symptoms, diminishing bodily preoccupation, distress, depression, and anxiety, and significantly increase control over one's thoughts and behaviors, and improve functioning. In some cases, they are lifesaving.

To Contact The Body Image Program At Butler Hospital

The Body Image Program
Butler Hospital
345 Blackstone Boulevard
Providence, RI 02906
Phone: 401-455-6466 or 401-455-6613
Website: http://www.butler.org/bdd.html

Cognitive-behavioral therapy is a here-and-now type of therapy in which the therapist helps the person with BDD resist compulsive BDD behaviors (for example, mirror checking) and face avoided situations (for example, social situations). It's important to determine whether a therapist has been specifically trained in cognitive-behavioral therapy. Other types of treatment (for example, counseling or psychotherapy) do not appear to be effective when used alone for BDD.

For More Information About BDD

- *The Broken Mirror: Understanding and Treating Body Dysmorphic Disorder* by Katharine A. Phillips, M.D. (Director of the Body Image Program), Oxford University Press, 1998 (ISBN: 0195121260). This book is a comprehensive source of information on body dysmorphic disorder and is written for both professionals and people with BDD and their families.

- "Learning to Live With Body Dysmorphic Disorder," by Katharine A. Phillips, M.D., Barbara Livingstone Van Noppen, M.S.W., and Leslie Shapiro, M.S.W.. This document is a booklet written for family members of individuals with body dysmorphic disorder. This booklet can be obtained for a charge plus $2 for shipping and handling from the Obsessive Compulsive Foundation, 337 Notch Hill Road, North Branford, CT 06471; Phone: 203-315-2190; Fax: 203-315-2196; Website: http://www.ocfoundation.org. Contact the Obsessive Compulsive Foundation for current pricing and availability.

- Information on body dysmorphic disorder can also be obtained from professional journals. These journals can be located through Medline (the bibliographic database of the National Library of Medicine, a primary source of biomedical information) and PsycLit (a database of international literature in psychology and related behavioral and social sciences). These databases are accessible at most university, college, and medical school libraries.

Chapter 33

Self-Injury

Frequently Asked Questions About Self-Injury

What Is Self-Injury?

Self-injury (SI) is the act of physically hurting yourself on purpose without the intent of committing suicide. It is a method of coping during an emotionally difficult time that helps some people temporarily feel better because they have a way to physically express and release the tension and the pain they hold inside. In other people hurting themselves produces chemical changes in their bodies that make them feel happier and more relaxed.

Five key components identify and define SI.

- One, SI is a harmful act done to yourself. Do not mistake lashing out in anger at others as SI.

- Two, SI is only done by yourself. If anyone else does something to you that causes pain this is not SI.

- Three, an act of SI must include some sort of physical violence. Emotionally punishing yourself (calling yourself a bitch or thinking you're stupid, ugly, etc.) is not SI.

About This Chapter: Text in this chapter was excerpted and adapted with permission from www.self-injury.net; reviewed by David A. Cooke, M.D., March 4, 2001.

• Four, an act of SI is not done with the intention of killing yourself. People who slit their wrists to kill themselves, even though they have harmed their body, are not SI-ing.

• Last, SI is done intentionally—not accidentally, but with the intent of hurting yourself.

Who Typically Takes Part In SI?

• *Gender:* Both men and women hurt themselves. More often women are seen with this behavior in a therapist's office, a psychiatric hospital, etc. Whereas more men are seen with SI in prisons.

• *Age:* SI behavior usually begins when a person is a teenager, escalates in a person's twenties, and disappears by their thirties.

> ✤ **It's A Fact!!**
>
> ## What About Tattooing And Body Piercing?
>
> Behaviors that alter the appearance of the body are generally used to make the person look better. In SI this is rarely, if ever, the case. Also, SI and body alteration are done by different methods. While SI is done by yourself, body alteration is typically done by another—usually someone who is licensed and/or trained.

• *Substance Abuse:* Many people who SI have histories of drug and alcohol abuse. Often this is because drugs are another method of coping because they can temporarily ease internal pain. But rarely are people under the influence when they SI.

• *Eating Disorders:* Eating disorders, such as anorexia or bulimia, are common in people who hurt themselves. Like SI, eating disorders often have the same psychological effects. Sometimes SI and eating disorders occur simultaneously.

• *History of Abuse:* The majority of people who hurt themselves have suffered physical, sexual, or emotional abuse. But this doesn't mean that everyone who SIs has been abused. Or that everybody who has been abused will start hurting themselves.

What Ways Do People SI?

SI is usually split into three categories: Psychotic, Organic, and Typical.

- **Psychotic SI:** Types of Psychotic SI include the removal or amputation of body parts, such as eyes, limbs, ears, and genitals. These acts of SI are usually done in response to visual or audible hallucinations. This type of SI is severe and is easily identified.

- **Organic SI:** Organic SI usually stems from autistic disorders, developmental disabilities, and other psychologically induced disorders. This type of SI is always influenced by physical or chemical problems in the body. Forms of Organic SI include head-banging and lip-biting.

- **Typical SI:** Typical SI results because of emotional or psychological reasons not related to psychotic (hearing voices, seeing things that aren't there, delusions) or organic (physical) conditions. The majority of the people who SI fall into this category. This type of SI is used to make yourself feel better and as a way of coping with your life. The following are the most common ways people hurt themselves.

  - *Cutting:* Cutting, also known as slicing or slashing, is the most common way people hurt themselves. It is typically done with a knife, razor blade, piece of glass, or other sharp objects. Most of the cuts are done on the arms, legs, wrists, and chest; but other people cut on other parts of the body such as the stomach, face, neck, breasts, and genitals. But cutting on the arms and wrist is the most common because excuses can be made more easily (for example people can say that they had an accident while cooking).

  - *Burning:* Burning is another common way people hurt themselves. Usually done with cigarettes, lighters, matches, kitchen-stove burners, heated objects (branding irons or hot skillets), and burning objects. Sometimes people even use flammable substances such as gasoline, propane, alcohol, and lighter fluid. Similar to cutting, most people burn themselves on their arms, wrists, legs, and chest.

  - *Interference with the Healing of Wounds:* Most people have unconsciously interfered with the healing of a wound but it is considered

SI when it is done deliberately. Some people remove stitches prematurely, stick objects such as needles, pins, etc. into the wound, or do other things to re-open the wound.

- *Hitting:* Another way that people hurt themselves is hitting themselves with their fists, most commonly done on the head or thighs. Although it may not seem as serious as cutting or burning it is done for the same reasons and results.

- *Extreme Nail Biting:* It is common for most people to bite their nails. But when it is used as a form of SI it is more severe and frequent than normal. It can result in the injury and damage of the fingernails or cuticles. People can bite their fingernails so much that they draw blood.

- *Scratching:* Scratching can become a form of SI. People who use it as a method of SI make it more extreme in frequency, intensity, and duration. Areas of skin can become raw

✎ Weird Words

Diagnostic and Statistical Manual IV (DSM-IV): Complete title of this book, which is produced by the American Psychiatric Association, is *Diagnostic and Statistical Manual of Mental Disorders, Fourth Edition.* It provides standard names and descriptions of mental disorders; these terms and guidelines are used by health care providers in making diagnostic assessments. The first edition was published in 1952; the fourth edition, which is the most recent, was published in 1994.

Dissociation: The separation of normal thought processes from the conscious mind. An extreme example of dissociation is multiple personality disorder (also called dissociative identity disorder), in which a person exhibits two or more distinct conscious personalities.

Organic: Having to do with the structure or chemicals of the body.

Psychotic: Associated with psychosis, which is the loss of contact with reality, delusions, or hallucinations.

Rituals: Activities or other routines that are performed compulsively and repeatedly to relieve or prevent anxiety.

or sometimes even bloody. Usually the scratching is done with the fingernails but sometimes it is done with a sharp or semisharp object such as a knife, comb, or pencil. Sometimes it is done unconsciously.

- *Hair-Pulling:* Trichotillomania, "the excessive and recurrent removal of your own hair resulting in a noticeable loss of hair," is the only form of SI recognized as a psychological disorder by the *Diagnostic and Statistical Manual of Mental Disorders (DSM-IV)*. Usually the hair is removed from the scalp, eyebrows, or beard, but can be from any part of the body. The bald spots that result from trichotillomania are usually covered with a hat, bandage, or sunglasses.

- *Breaking of Bones:* A form of SI that is more rare than the others, the breaking of bones is a serious and severe form of SI. Usually, people break their bones with an instrument such as a hammer, brick, or other heavy objects. But sometimes people throw themselves into walls or doors.

Why Would Anybody Intentionally Hurt Themselves?

Often people hurt themselves to try to relieve intense emotions and feel better. These intense feelings can seem uncontrollable, frightening, and dangerous. When people have them they may think that hurting themselves is the only way to escape these feelings.

People who hurt themselves often are unable to control their emotions. They cannot experience and express them the way most people do: by crying, screaming, yelling, etc.

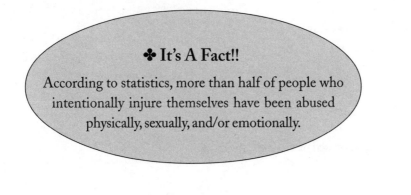

♣ It's A Fact!!
According to statistics, more than half of people who intentionally injure themselves have been abused physically, sexually, and/or emotionally.

Therapy For Self-Injury

If you do decide to enter therapy, be aware that this is not a magical solution to your problems. You will not go to therapy and be instantly "cured." Therapy requires motivation and commitment to be helpful. Therefore, your decision to enter therapy should be given a lot of thought.

Finding A Good Therapist

Once you have decided to enter therapy, you will need to find a therapist. It is generally easy to locate a therapist, but it is more difficult to find a therapist who is well qualified and suited to your particular needs. You may be able to locate a therapist through a referral from a friend, family member, physician, or someone else who knows you well. You will generally have better luck finding a good therapist through a referral than you would through an advertisement or the yellow pages. But regardless of how you find the therapist's name and telephone number, you should ask some questions before entering therapy with that individual.

Because therapy involves such an intense and personal relationship between the therapist and the client, it is important that you find a therapist you are comfortable with. You level of comfort may be influenced by many factors,

> ### ✔ Quick Tip
>
> The following questions will help you in your search to find a therapist:
>
> - What type of degree and/or license do you have?
>
> - How much experience do you have in treating self-injury?
>
> - What is the normal course of treatment for self-injury?
>
> - How much do you know about areas related to self-injury (such as trauma, abuse, eating disorders, dissociation, or dissociative disorders?
>
> - How long do you expect I'll be in therapy?
>
> - What is your general availability?
>
> - How much do you charge?
>
> - Is there anything else that you think I should know about you or the way you do therapy?

including the therapist's academic degree, knowledge, psychotherapeutic approach, age, sex, experience, and personality.

What Happens In Therapy?

The experiences of each person in therapy will be different, because what happens in therapy depends on you. How you choose to use each session, your particular therapist's approach and experience, and your own knowledge, experience, and motivation will help determine your therapy.

In the majority of cases, the first few therapeutic sessions will be spent relating historical or factual information and developing or defining therapeutic goals. During these first sessions you are getting to know your therapist, and vice versa, and determining whether this therapeutic relationship will suit your particular needs.

After these first few sessions is when the real work begins. Your perceptions of therapy and your therapist will most likely fluctuate, as well as your commitment to therapy. All of these experiences are normal and to be expected.

How To Stop Hurting Yourself

After you have decided it is the time to stop hurting yourself, you need to answer the question of how. There are many different methods to help you in stopping or reducing self-injury behaviors in the short-term—at the time you feel the need or desire to hurt yourself. But, first, it is important to examine some long-term approaches.

Changing Your Behaviors

When you change your behaviors, you change the organization of your thoughts, feelings, and physical sensations. This means that by changing the behaviors associated with self-injury you will alter the frequency of and the way in which you engage in hurting yourself. You will also alter some of the fundamental reasons for self-injury.

- *Time and Place.* Some people have a particular time of day when they are more likely to engage in self-injury. It is important that you monitor and assess when you are more likely to hurt yourself. If you change the pattern of your activities during these times, you can lessen the chance that you will hurt yourself.

- *Means.* Getting rid of any instruments that you usually use to hurt yourself is another important change. You should do this before you feel the desire to hurt yourself. If you use a knife, throw it away. Or if you use matches, throw them away. You may not be able to bring yourself to get rid of these objects. In this case, then put them in a box and hide it under something heavy or difficult to move. Basically, make whatever instruments you usually use to hurt yourself as inaccessible as possible. By doing this you will make it more difficult for you to hurt yourself, which lessens the chance that you will actually do so.

- *Rituals.* Another way to change your behaviors is to alter the patterns or rituals associated with self-injury. Changing a part of your self-injury ritual will make SI more uncomfortable and less reinforcing for you. The less comfortable you feel when you are hurting yourself, the less likely you are to engage in your self-injurious behavior. Changing your routines also makes you more aware of your surroundings and of your behaviors. This awareness can conflict with dissociation and therefore can reduce self-injury.

Getting Support

It is essential to reduce feelings of isolation and alienation because the desire for self-injury often stems from these feelings. Most people hurt themselves when they are alone. You are less likely to hurt yourself if you place yourself in situations where other people are present.

When you feel the need to hurt yourself, call a friend. Or call more than one friend. Have another person come and sit with you, or go and sit with someone else. Use the support systems you have formed.

Another simple and effective method of changing an unwanted behavior is based on one rule: "Never engage in any activity unless you are able to tell at least two people of your plans." If you are unable to do this, it is likely that it is not a good thing for you to do. This rule can apply to many things, including self-injury.

Changing Your Thoughts

Another part of ending or reducing self-injurious behavior is to change the thoughts you have regarding them. The thoughts that occur before an act of self-injury are largely responsible for your desire and decision to hurt yourself. Because of the power of these thoughts, it is very important that you break this cycle and change your thoughts before you engage in an act of self-injury.

You most likely have many negative thoughts before you hurt yourself. You may accept the thoughts that pass through your mind as true, but this is often not the case. A good way to change your negative thoughts is to challenge their accuracy. It is important that you question each negative thought you have been able to identify. It is better for you to stop or change your negative thoughts than to permit yourself to continue negative and potentially dangerous styles of thoughts.

✔ Quick Tip

You can change your negative thoughts into positive ones. For example:

Negative Thought	Positive Thought
"I'm so dumb for hurting myself."	"I did what I needed to do to take care of myself."
"I can't believe I let myself do this again."	"I used the best method possible at that time to cope."
"I have to keep this a secret."	"I can decide who I would like to tell—and not to tell—about this."

Changing Your Feelings

It is important that you realize the difference between change and denial. It is very dangerous to fail to recognize emotions that you are feeling or to pretend that they do not exist. Usually, expressing your emotions and acting on them is a highly effective way of dealing with feelings—much more effective than pretending that they do not exist or ignoring them.

The first step you must take to change your emotions is to learn to identify what you are feeling. You may be using self-injury as a way to express or regulate your feelings. But you may be unaware of what emotions produce an episode of self-injury. The ability to identify specific feelings is necessary for attempting to change them.

Once you have begun learning to identify your emotions the easiest way to change them is by expressing them. Feelings are hard to ignore but if you express them, they will be satisfied. Each feeling has its own method of expression. It will take a lot of practice and patience to find the match between your feelings and the best way to express them.

The majority of the feelings you have will require some type of physical release. Crying is a simple example of this release. Learning to identify and express your feelings will gradually cause your feelings to change. And this change will allow you to feel more content and resolved. But, withholding, denying, or avoiding your feelings will increase the chances of wanting to hurt yourself.

Self-injury may have been your way of releasing your emotions. And while in the past this may have been effective and necessary, you may find that other ways of expressing your emotions work just as good and have less negative consequences.

Changing Your Physical Sensations

The body and mind affect each other. Physical problems affect psychological problems, and vice versa. The way in which you treat your body affects your psychological health, so when you hurt yourself, you are also hurting your psychological health. But if you take care of your body, your psychological health will profit.

You can train your body to produce different physical behaviors and sensations. Before you hurt yourself you most likely feel a great state of tension. And at this time it may seem that SI is the best or only way to reduce this tension. But there are other options that will produce similar results and are less physically damaging.

A simple way to change your physical sensations is to exercise. Exercising increases your heart rate and changes other physical patterns such as respiration, digestion, and blood flow. It can also alter the exchange of neurotransmitters in your brain. These chemical neurotransmitters in your brain influence your physical experience.

It is important that you identify the type of physical exercise you enjoy as well as how convenient or accessible they are to you. Try to think of as many options as you can that will allow you to exercise when you feel the urge to hurt yourself.

Talking To Other People About Self-Injury

A majority of the things we do affect others, whether we intend them to or not. Even "nonbehaviors" can affect other people. For example, not showing up when someone expects you makes a strong statement. Our facial expressions, body language, tone of voice, silence, and actions all can affect the reactions and behaviors of other people. The behavior and "nonbehavior" of others affects us as well.

When you tell loved ones that you are purposely inflicted injury on yourself, they are most likely going to have some strong reactions. The following section will discuss the a few of the most common reactions and how you can overcome their negative effects.

Self-Injury Keeps Other People At A Distance

Self-injury encourages emotional distance for other people in several ways. You may have not told anyone about your self-injury. You may edit information about your behaviors and how you feel (your emotional states.) You may even lie about what you do and how you feel. Each of these impairs or severs communication and intimacy with other people, which creates distance. You can't be close with others if you are dishonest with them.

Dissociation that may come with self-injury may also create emotional distance. Remember that dissociation may come before or after an act of self-injury. You cannot feel connected with other people if you are in a dissociated state, because during dissociation you feel disconnected from yourself. You can't feel emotionally close to other people if you are distant from yourself.

Coping With Other People's Reactions To Your SI

It is very important to realize how much your actions affect others around you. Self-injury causes many different emotions and reactions in others. You may not have the intention of provoking a reaction, you may not even want others to know about your SI, but most likely the will react.

Most of the reactions others have to your self-injury will be negative. You may have already noticed this if you have noticeable scars or wounds. People may see people staring at your scars or wounds, or hear cruel remarks on your mental state. Also, other people may treat you differently after they find out about your self-injurious activities.

You may experience negative reactions to your self-injury, if you have not already. And you may be unprepared for these reactions. You may be so focused on the great amount of courage and effort it takes to tell others about your SI, that the possible ramifications for others may not have occurred to you. Eventually you will notice some of the negative effects of telling others about your SI. You possibly may lose friends because they are unable or unwilling to deal with your self-injurious behavior. There may be subtler changes in your relationships with others, such as friends or family members inspecting you for new injuries. Also, friends and family may focus your conversations on your SI rather than other parts of your life. Each of these reactions will change your relationship in some way.

Another reaction which is one of the most difficult and damaging is nonreaction. Sometimes others will not respond to your behaviors, which may make you feel invisible. When you are ignored, the feelings of being invisible can lead to feelings of isolation and alienation that are part of the SI cycle.

It would be nice to not be affected by the reactions of others, but this is not likely to happen. Whatever the other person's reaction, it will almost certainly have an impact on you. On method you may use to cope with others reactions is to try to understand why they are reacting this way. Since you can't control others reactions, you can only try to understand them.

Learning To Communicate Directly

Self-injury is a very indirect method of communication. And the message that others receive why they learn about your self-injurious behavior likely will be distorted and inaccurate. You may think that your SI only communicates one message, but it actually send many, some of which may not be what you intended. This is miscommunication.

Miscommunication has many results. First, your needs will be left unmet because you are unlikely to get your point across. Also, SI is often misinterpreted as an act of manipulation. Because self-injury is an indirect form of communication, people might think that you are trying to provoke a response or reaction from them. In some cases this may be true, but most often, manipulation is not the goal of SI.

Instead of using self-injury as a form of communication, it would be better to talk about self-injury directly with other people. Messages you are trying to transmit will be communicated much more clearly with words than with self-injury.

☞ **Remember!!**

Self-injury is method of coping some people use during emotionally difficult times. For more information about self injury and the healing process, visit the Self-Injury Network at www.self-injury.net.

Chapter 34

Delusions And Delusional Disorders

Delusions are a common symptom of many illnesses and mental abnormalities and the unique, defining feature of one type of psychiatric condition, the delusional disorders. As described in the American Psychiatric Association's diagnostic manual, these disorders consist of delusions persisting for at least a month with no known organic cause and no other obvious mental or emotional disorder or medical condition. The delusions are not bizarre, that is, not totally implausible by the standards of the culture.

The Five Types Of Delusional Disorder

Five types of delusional disorder are listed in the manual. Most common are delusions of persecution—the belief that you are under attack, often the target of a conspiracy. You are being harassed, threatened, cheated, spied on, ridiculed, followed, or poisoned. Delusions of jealousy have a lover's infidelity as their theme. Erotomania (also known as de Clerembault's syndrome) is the delusion that someone is in love with you—usually someone of higher social status, often a stranger, and sometimes a celebrity. People with delusions of grandeur may believe that they are unrecognized geniuses, can banish poverty and ensure world peace, or have been chosen by God as messengers

About This Chapter: The text in this chapter is from "Delusions and Delusional Disorders," excerpted from the January 1999 issue of the *Harvard Mental Health Letter*, © 1999, by the President and Fellow of Harvard College; reprinted with permission.

to humanity. The body is the center of somatic delusions: you believe that you are emitting a horrible smell or have an intestinal parasite, or that some body part is ugly or deformed or not functioning properly.

The reasoning of people with delusional disorders is not necessarily flawed in any obvious way, and the resulting system of beliefs may be elaborately plausible and even superficially convincing. They rarely have hallucinations,

✎ Weird Words

Capgras' Syndrome: A delusional belief that a family member or close friend has been replaced by an imposter.

Delusion: A false belief or wrong judgement about reality maintained despite contradictory evidence or logic. Some specific delusions are: *delusion of grandeur*—an exaggerated belief in one's own importance, wealth, or power; *delusions of persecution*—a belief that one is being systematically victimized by other people; *delusions of control*—a belief that one's thoughts and actions are being imposed by an outside force; *nihilistic delusion*—a belief that the world has ceased to exist; and *somatic delusions*—a belief that something is wrong with the body.

Erotomania: A type of delusion in which a person believes he or she is involved in a loving relationship with another person, such as someone who is famous or who is not available for social reasons.

Hypochondria: A persistent preoccupation with one's health and fear of having a disease despite assurances and physical evidence of health; exaggerated attention toward physical and mental symptoms.

Obsession: A mental state characterized by a persistent, recurring, unwanted idea, often one that is recognized as senseless, but that cannot be eliminated.

Psychosis: A severe mental illness of organic or emotional origin which is characterized by a loss of contact with reality, delusions, or hallucinations. Psychosis causes a distortion of a person's mental processes and interferes with ordinary activities and relationships of daily life.

and their personalities do not change. Although the consequences of their delusions can be serious—social isolation, rejection, stalking, harassment, and violence—they usually come to the attention of lawyers or plastic surgeons before they seek the help of mental health professionals.

Other Forms Of Delusion

Of course, delusions take many other forms besides these five. In schizophrenia, the most serious common brain disease of early adulthood, delusions are usually not well organized and well reasoned, but fragmentary and confused (reflecting the schizophrenic thought disorder) and bizarre (reflecting the strangeness of schizophrenic experience). A delusion typical of schizophrenia and other psychotic disorders is the belief that thoughts are being inserted into one's head or broadcast to the world. Psychotically depressed persons may believe that they are being punished in hell or that the world has been annihilated. The elation and hyperactive thought processes of manic patients often produce delusions of grandeur or persecution.

Another disorder with prominent delusions is late paraphrenia, a poorly understood condition that occurs mainly in old age. Its symptoms consist of delusions and hallucinations that resemble schizophrenia, without the disordered thinking and emotional unresponsiveness of schizophrenic patients. Late paraphrenia probably has many causes including deafness, social isolation, slowly developing brain disease, and unrecognized infarcts (strokes). Delusions are also a common symptom of dementia in all its forms and a common effect of physical illnesses, including endocrine and metabolic disorders, multiple sclerosis, chronic liver disease, pernicious anemia, and migraine. Another fertile source is drug intoxication and withdrawal—especially alcoholic hallucinosis and alcohol withdrawal delirium (which produces shifting, confused delusions) and acute and chronic abuse of amphetamines and cocaine (in which the delusions are sometimes well organized and persistent).

What Is A Delusion?

Although we often speak as though everyone can recognize a pathological delusion, there is no simple definition or identifying sign. In the glossary of the APA's diagnostic manual, a delusion is defined as a false personal belief based on an incorrect inference about external reality, rejected by others in one's own culture, that is firmly maintained in contradiction to the beliefs of others and despite obvious and irrefutable proof or evidence to the contrary. Critics of this definition say that the reasoning involved in a delusion is not necessarily wrong, and the reality at which it is directed may be internal. Many ideas that turn out to be correct are first maintained despite nearly universal skepticism. In daily life we do not act like scientists, continually testing the correspondence of our thoughts with reality. Many beliefs—most religious doctrines, for example—cannot be tested at all. Many others are acquired by incorrect inferences, indoctrination, and custom. Delusions may be temporary rather than fixed, and many ordinary beliefs are stubbornly maintained despite contrary evidence. A delusion can even make itself come true; for example, a belief in malicious witchcraft may cause a depression or psychosis that ends in death.

Delusions Vs. Obsessions

As the diagnostic manual acknowledges, a delusion may also be difficult to distinguish from an obsessional thought that is no longer resisted and becomes an "overvalued idea." In one study, nearly 50% of patients with obsessive-compulsive disorder were certain or nearly certain that if they did not perform their compulsive rituals, some harm would come to them. The line between obsession and delusion is also difficult to draw in body dysmorphic disorder, an irrational anxiety about imagined ugliness, and hypochondriasis, the interpretation of minor physical symptoms as signs of serious illness. In the end, social acceptability usually determines what is

♣ It's A Fact!!

The five most common forms of delusional disorders are:

- Delusions of persecution

- Delusions of jealousy

- Delusions that someone is in love with the patient (called "erotomania")

- Delusions of grandeur

- Somatic delusions (the belief that something is wrong with the patient's body)

treated as a delusion rather than merely an idiosyncratic, unpersuasive, superstitious, or overvalued false idea.

Delusions arise from experiences, external or internal, that are felt to be unusual, significant, and urgently in need of explanation. A strange feeling, perception, or persistent thought occurs, and the person affected needs to make sense of it—above all, to understand why it is happening to him or her and not to others. A delusional interpretation, however disturbing it may be and however damaging in the long run, provides immediate relief, just as performing a compulsive ritual brings relief from an obsessional thought. Unless the delusion is associated with a general deterioration of brain functions, as in schizophrenia or dementia, it is compatible with adequate and even superior thinking. Once the delusion is well established, apparently contrary evidence can easily be ignored or accommodated.

The raw material is supplied by many kinds of experiences: hallucinatory odors, visions, and voices, an unexplained feeling or absence of feeling, or a sensory defect, emotional state, or social situation that makes communication difficult and promotes suspicion. The stranger the experience, the more bizarre the explanation. Schizophrenic patients hear voices issuing commands or sense that their thoughts are somehow not their own, and they try to still their anxiety by identifying the external power that is controlling their minds. The experiences that form the basis of delusional disorders are more common and the resulting delusions less obviously implausible.

Delusional Misidentification

In most cases, character, social circumstances, and past experience determine the nature of the delusion—how a person interprets the unusual experience. But certain brain malfunctions can produce highly characteristic delusions that are not affected by any of these influences. A striking example is delusional misidentification. This phenomenon has many possible causes (including schizophrenia, mood disorders, dementia, and alcohol abuse), but it sometimes occurs, like delusional disorders, in the apparent absence of any other medical or psychiatric symptoms. The most common form is the Capgras syndrome—a belief, often difficult or impossible to shake, that certain important people have been replaced by nearly identical duplicates. A man with the Capgras delusion may insist, for example, that his wife has gone away and her place has been taken by someone who looks just like her, or even by a robot.

The disorder has many variants, including the Fregoli delusion (someone you know is taking on the appearance of other people), reduplicative paramnesia (you have another self, or your original self has been replaced), and intermetamorphosis (others are mistaking you for someone else or you have exchanged identities with someone else). In a related condition, Cotard's syndrome, patients may say that they are dead or no longer exist or that their brains are missing. A surprisingly common delusion is the denial of paralysis: a person whose left side is immobilized by a stroke calmly insists that she can move the left arm and leg—or sometimes, even more bizarrely, that the paralyzed limb is not her own, although it is attached to her body.

✔ Quick Tip

The following articles and books can give you more information about delusional disorders.

For Further Reading

Brad A. Alford and Aaron T. Beck. "Cognitive therapy of delusional beliefs." *Behavioural Research and Therapy* 32(3): 369-380 (1994).

"Delusional disorders." *Psychiatric Clinics of North America* 18(2) (June 1995).

Brendan A. Maher and Manfred Spitzer. "Delusions." In: Patricia B. Sutker and Henry E. Adams, eds. *Comprehensive Handbook of Psychopathology, Second Edition*. New York: Plenum Press, 1993.

V.S. Ramachandran and Sandra Blakeslee. *Phantoms in the Brain*. New York: William Morrow, 1998.

Observers of these delusions have repeatedly looked for a motive, conscious or unconscious. There are obvious reasons for not wanting to admit being paralyzed. A patient with the Capgras syndrome may say that the replacement is somehow different from the original—usually less loving and considerate. One's own double is often older than one's "real" self. Psychoanalysts have suggested an explanation for both the doubling and the difference. In infancy we regard our parents in turn as entirely good and entirely bad, generous fairies or wicked witches.

> **☞ Remember!!**
>
> There are many types of delusions. The reasoning of people with delusional disorders is not necessarily flawed in any obvious way, and the resulting system of beliefs may be elaborately plausible and even superficially convincing.

Eventually we learn how to live with ambivalent feelings about the people we love, and the good and bad parents become one person. Under stress we may regress emotionally, returning to the infantile state in which we are free to love the good, "real" parent and hate the evil impostor.

But people with misidentification delusions do not always respond in ways that would be natural if these explanations were generally right. The duplicate is not necessarily hated or feared. Asked to explain why his mother and father have been replaced, a patient may look puzzled and suggest that they have hired the substitutes to look after him. Besides, people may say that not only family members but favorite pets have been duplicated. As for patients who deny paralysis, they rarely seem anxious or defensive, as though they are trying to hide something from themselves. A person with a paralyzed arm, asked to clap her hands, may be satisfied by the sound of one hand clapping against the air. Or she may make an implausible casual excuse for not moving the arm: "I have arthritis, and my shoulder hurts"; "I'm tired of having all these medical students prodding me." In Cotard's syndrome, the feeling of being dead does not always inspire the appropriate despair or terror; these patients may even talk of their supposedly rotting flesh without apparent emotion. And it is hard to see how an unconscious motive can explain why all these delusions are so often associated with a specific kind of brain damage—injury to the right hemisphere of the cerebral cortex.

Chapter 35

Schizophrenia

Schizophrenia is a serious biological brain disorder which affects how a person thinks, feels and acts. Someone with schizophrenia has difficulty distinguishing between what is real and what is imaginary; is often unresponsive or withdrawn; and has difficulty expressing normal emotions in social situations.

Schizophrenia is a misunderstood disease. It is not split personality or multiple personality, but rather a "shattered" personality. The vast majority of its sufferers are not violent and do not pose a danger to others. Schizophrenia is not caused by childhood experiences, poor parenting or lack of willpower, nor are the symptoms identical for each person.

What Causes Schizophrenia?

The theories about the cause of schizophrenia are numerous and complex. Several of the more widely accepted theories about the cause of this disease include: genetics (heredity), biology, (the imbalance in the brain's chemistry); and/or possible viral infections and immune disorders. However, it is not clear if one or all of these theories are factors in causing the disease.

About This Chapter: The text in this chapter is from "Schizophrenia: What You Need to Know," produced by the National Mental Health Association in July 1997 and updated in October 1999, and supported by an educational grant from Eli Lilly and Company, © National Mental Health Association. Reprinted with permission from the National Mental Health Association (1-800-969-NMHA).

Genetics (Heredity)

Scientists recognize that the disorder tends to run in families and that a person inherits a tendency to develop the disease. Schizophrenia may be triggered by environmental events, such as viral infections or highly stressful situations or a combination of both.

Similar to some other genetically related illnesses, schizophrenia appears when the body undergoes hormonal and physical changes, like those that occur during puberty in the teen and young adult years.

Chemistry

Genetics help to determine how the brain uses certain chemicals. People with schizophrenia have a chemical imbalance of brain chemicals (serotonin and dopamine) which are neurotransmitters. These neurotransmitters allow nerve cells in the brain to send messages to each other. The imbalance of these chemicals affects the way a person's brain reacts to stimuli—which explains why a person with schizophrenia may be overwhelmed by sensory information (loud music or bright lights) which other people can easily handle. This problem in processing different sounds, sights, smells and tastes can also lead to hallucinations or delusions.

✤ It's A Fact!!

Schizophrenia— Who's Likely To Suffer From It?

Schizophrenia affects about 1% of the world population. In the United States, about 2.5 million people have this disease, about one in a hundred people.

Symptoms usually appear between the ages of 13 and 25, but often appear earlier in males than females.

What Are The Symptoms Of Schizophrenia?

The signs of schizophrenia are different for everyone. Symptoms may develop slowly over months or years, or may appear very abruptly. The disease may come and go in cycles of relapse and remission.

Behaviors that may be early warning signs of schizophrenia include:

- Hearing or seeing something that isn't there.
- A constant feeling of being watched.
- Peculiar or nonsensical way of speaking or writing.
- Strange posturing.
- Feeling indifferent to very important situations.
- Deterioration of academic or work performance.
- A change in personal hygiene and appearance.
- A change in personality.
- Increasing withdrawal from social situations.
- Irrational, angry, or fearful response to loved ones.
- Inability to sleep or concentrate.
- Inappropriate or bizarre behavior.
- Extreme preoccupation with religion or the occult.

> ✎ **Weird Words**
>
> <u>Remission:</u> A lessening in the severity of a disease evidenced by the elimination or reduction of symptoms. Remission also describes the period of time during which disease symptoms are abated.
>
> <u>Schizophrenia:</u> A class of mental illnesses marked by abnormalities in perception, changes in mood and behavior, withdrawal from other people and the outside world, and disturbances of thinking, including misinterpretation of reality, delusions, and hallucinations.

If you or a loved one experience many of these symptoms for more than two weeks, seek medical help immediately.

Positive And Negative Symptoms

Positive symptoms are disturbances that are "added" to the person's personality

- Delusions—false ideas—individuals may believe that someone is spying on him or her, or that they are someone famous.

- Hallucinations—imaginary voices which give commands or comments to the individual. It is less common for the person to think he or she sees, feels, tastes, or smells something which really doesn't exist.

- Disordered thinking—moving from one topic to another, but making no sense. Individuals may make up their own words or sounds.

Negative symptoms are capabilities that are "lost" from the person's personality.

- Social withdrawal
- Extreme apathy
- Lack of drive or initiative
- Emotional unresponsiveness

What Are The Different Types Of Schizophrenia?

- Paranoid schizophrenia—a person feels extremely suspicious, persecuted, grandiose, or experiences a combination of these emotions.

- Disorganized schizophrenia—a person is often incoherent but may not have delusions.

- Catatonic schizophrenia—a person is withdrawn, mute, negative and often assumes very unusual postures.

- Residual schizophrenia—a person is no longer experiencing delusions or hallucinations,

✔ Quick Tip

Coping Guidelines For The Caretakers Of The Person With Schizophrenia

1. Help the person stay on the medication.

2. Establish a daily routine for the person to follow.

3. Keep the lines of communication open about problems or fears the person may have.

4. Understand that caring for the person can be emotionally and physically exhausting. Take time for yourself.

5. Keep your communications simple and brief when speaking with the person.

6. Be patient and calm.

7. Ask for help if you need it; join a support group.

but has no motivation or interest in fife. These symptoms can be most devastating.

• Schizoaffective disorder—a person has symptoms of both schizophrenia and a major mood disorder such as depression.

What Treatments Are Available For Schizophrenia?

If you suspect someone you know is experiencing symptoms of schizophrenia, encourage them to see a psychiatrist immediately. Early treatment— even as early as the first episode—can mean a higher remission rate and a better long-term outcome.

Antipsychotic Drugs

Schizophrenia is usually a lifelong disease. Most people with this illness will probably take medication for the rest of their lives, as do people with diabetes, high blood pressure or heart disease.

Antipsychotic medications help to normalize the biochemical imbalances that cause schizophrenia. They are also important in reducing the likelihood of relapse. Like all medications, however, antipsychotic drugs should be taken only under close supervision of a psychiatrist or other physician.

There are two major types of medications: conventional antipsychotics and the new generation of antipsychotics introduced in the 1990s called atypical antipsychotics.

Conventional antipsychotics effectively control the "positive" symptoms such as hallucinations, delusions, and confusion of schizophrenia.

Atypical antipsychotics treat both the "positive" and "negative" symptoms of schizophrenia with fewer side effects.

Side effects are common with antipsychotic drugs. Traditional antipsychotic drugs have side effects that range from mild side effects such as dry mouth, blurred vision, constipation, drowsiness and dizziness which usually disappear after a few weeks to more serious side effects such as trouble with muscle control, pacing, tremors and facial ticks. The newer generation of drugs, the atypicals, have fewer side effects. However, it is important to talk with your doctor before making any changes in medication since many side effects can be controlled.

Counseling And Rehabilitation

Rehabilitation can help a person regain the confidence to take care of themselves and live a fuller fife. Different forms of "talk" therapy, both individual and group, can help both the patient and family members to better understand the illness and share their coping problems.

About This Chapter

This text was reviewed by:

David Shore, MD, Acting Deputy Director, Division of Clinical Research and Treatment Research, National Institute of Mental Health.

J. R. Elpers, MD, Department of Psychiatry, Harbor-UCL4 Medical Center

Anne Brown, Director of Communications and Education, National Alliance for Research on Schizophrenia and Depression

Sources

The Harvard Mental Health Letter Schizophrenia: The Present State of Understanding Parts I and II, The Harvard Medical School, 74 Fernwood Road, Boston, MA 02115.

Understanding Schizophrenia: A Guide for People with Schizophrenia and their Families, National Alliance for Research on Schizophrenia and Depression (NARSAD), 1996.

"Essential Psychopathology and Its Treatment," by Jerrold S Maxmen and Nicholas G. Ward, Second edition, revised for *DSM-IV* 1995.

🖝 Remember!!

No cure for schizophrenia has been discovered, but with proper treatment, many people with this illness can lead productive and fulfilling lives.

For more information about schizophrenia, contact your local Mental Health Association or

National Mental Health Association
1021 Prince St.
Alexandria, VA 22314-2971
Toll-Free: 800-969-6642
Website: http://www.nmha.org

National Alliance for the Mentally Ill (NAMI)
2107 Wilson Blvd., Suite 300
Arlington, VA 22201
Toll-Free: 800-950-6264
Fax: 703-524-9094
Website: http://www.nami.org

National Alliance for Research on Schizophrenia and Depression (NARSAD)
60 Cutter Mill Road, Suite 404
Great Neck, NY 10021
Toll Free: 800-829-8289
Phone: 516-829-0091
Fax: 516-487-6930
Website: http://www.narsad.org
E-Mail: info@narsad.org

National Institute of Mental Health
6001 Executive Boulevard, Rm. 8184, MSC 9663
Rockville, MD 20892-9663
Toll-free 800-64-PANIC (647-2642)
Website: http://www.nimh.nih.gov

Part 3

Suicide

Chapter 36

Teenage Suicide

Most everyone at some time in his or her life will experience periods of anxiety, sadness, and despair. These are normal reactions to the pain of loss, rejection, or disappointment. Those with serious mental illnesses, however, often experience much more extreme reactions, reactions that can leave them mired in hopelessness. And when all hope is lost, some feel that suicide is the only solution. It isn't.

According to the National Institute of Mental Health, scientific evidence has shown that almost all people who take their own lives have a diagnosable mental or substance abuse disorder, and the majority have more than one disorder. In other words, the feelings that often lead to suicide are highly treatable. That's why it is imperative that we better understand the symptoms of the disorders and the behaviors that often accompany thoughts of suicide. With more knowledge, we can often prevent the devastation of losing a loved one.

Now the eighth-leading cause of death overall in the U.S. and the third-leading cause of death for young people between the ages of 15 and 24 years,

About This Chapter: Text in this chapter is from "Teenage Suicide," produced by the National Alliance for the Mentally Ill (NAMI) and reviewed by David Shaffer, M.D., F.R.C.P., F.R.C. Psych., Director, Department of Child Psychiatry, New York State Psychiatric Institute, Columbia College of Physicians and Surgeons, and Rex Cowdry, M.D., NAMI medical advisor, © 1999 NAMI. Reprinted with permission of the National Alliance for the Mentally Ill.

suicide has become the subject of much recent focus. U.S. Surgeon General David Satcher, for instance, announced his *Call to Action to Prevent Suicide*, 1999, an initiative intended to increase public awareness, promote intervention strategies, and enhance research. The media, too, has been paying very close attention to the subject of suicide, writing articles and books and running news stories. Suicide among our nation's youth, a population very vulnerable to self-destructive emotions, has perhaps received the most discussion of late. Maybe this is because teenage suicide seems the most tragic—lives lost before they've even started. Yet, while all of this recent focus is good, it's only the beginning. We cannot continue to lose so many lives unnecessarily.

It is a hopeful sign that while the incidence of suicide among adolescents and young adults nearly tripled from 1965 to 1987; teen suicide rates in the past ten years have actually been declining, possibly due to increased recognition and treatment. (1996 is the most recent year for which suicide statistics are available.)

Suicide "Signs"

There are many behavioral indicators that can help parents or friends recognize the threat of suicide in a loved one. Since mental and substance-related disorders so frequently accompany suicidal behavior, many of the cues to be looked for are symptoms associated with such disorders as depression, bipolar disorder (manic depression), anxiety disorders, alcohol and drug use, disruptive behavior disorders, borderline personality disorder, and schizophrenia.

Some common symptoms of these disorders include:

- Extreme personality changes
- Loss of interest in activities that used to be enjoyable
- Significant loss or gain in appetite
- Difficulty falling asleep or wanting to sleep all day
- Fatigue or loss of energy

- Feelings of worthlessness or guilt

- Withdrawal from family and friends

- Neglect of personal appearance or hygiene

- Sadness, irritability, or indifference

- Having trouble concentrating

- Extreme anxiety or panic

- Drug or alcohol use or abuse

- Aggressive, destructive, or defiant behavior

- Poor school performance

- Hallucinations or unusual beliefs

♣ **It's A Fact!!**

- In 1996, more teenagers and young adults died of suicide than from cancer, heart disease, AIDS, birth defects, stroke, pneumonia and influenza, and chronic lung disease combined.

- In 1996, suicide was the second-leading cause of death among college students, the third-leading cause of death among those aged 15 to 24 years, and the fourth-leading cause of death among those aged 10 to 14 years.

- From 1980 to 1996, the rate of suicide among African-American males aged 15 to 19 years increased by 105 percent.

Tragically, many of these signs go unrecognized. And while suffering from one of these symptoms certainly does not necessarily mean that one is suicidal, it's always best to communicate openly with a loved one who has one or more of these behaviors, especially if they are unusual for that person.

There are also some more obvious signs of the potential for committing suicide. Putting one's affairs in order, such as giving or throwing away favorite belongings, is a strong clue. And it can't be stressed more strongly that any talk of death or suicide should be taken seriously and paid close attention to. It is a sad fact that while many of those who commit suicide talked about it beforehand, only 33 percent to 50 percent were identified by their doctors as having a mental illness at the time of their death and only 15 percent of suicide victims were in treatment at the time of their death. Any history of previous suicide attempts is also reason for concern and watchfulness. Approximately one-third of teens who die by suicide have made a previous suicide attempt. It should be noted as well that while more females attempt suicide, more males are successful in completing suicide.

Causes

While the reasons that teens commit suicide vary widely, there are some common situations and circumstances that seem to lead to such extreme measures. These include major disappointment, rejection, failure, or loss such as breaking up with a girlfriend or boyfriend, failing a big exam, or witnessing family turmoil. Since the overwhelming majority of those who commit suicide have a mental or substance-related disorder, they often have difficulty coping with such crippling stressors. They are unable to see that their life can turn around, unable to recognize that suicide is a permanent solution to a temporary problem. Usually, the common reasons for suicide listed above are actually not the "causes" of the suicide, but rather triggers for suicide in a person suffering from a mental illness or substance-related disorder.

More recently, scientists have focused on the biology of suicide. Suicide is thought by some to have a genetic component, to run in families. And research has shown strong evidence that mental and substance-related disorders, which commonly affect those who end up committing suicide, do run in families. While the suicide of a relative is obviously not a direct "cause" of suicide, it does, perhaps, put certain individuals at more risk than others. Certainly, the suicide of one's parent or other close family member could lead to thoughts of such behavior in a teen with a mental or substance-related disorder.

Research has also explored the specific brain chemistry of those who take their own lives. Recent studies indicate that those who have attempted suicide may also have low levels of the brain chemical serotonin. Serotonin helps control impulsivity, and low levels of the brain chemical are thought to cause more impulsive behavior. Suicides are often committed out of impulse. Antidepressant drugs affecting serotonin are used to treat depression, impulsivity, and suicidal thoughts. However, much more research is needed to confirm these hypotheses and, hopefully, eventually lead to more definite indicators of and treatment for those prone to suicide.

How To Help

Since people who are contemplating suicide feel so alone and helpless, the most important thing to do if you think a friend or loved one is suicidal is to communicate with him or her openly and frequently. Make it clear that you care; stress your willingness to listen. Also, be sure to take all talk of suicide seriously. Don't assume that people who talk about killing themselves won't really do it. An estimated 80 percent of all those who commit suicide give some warning of their intentions or mention their feelings to a friend or family member. And don't ignore what may seem like casual threats or remarks. Statements like "You'll be sorry when I'm dead" and "I can't see any way out," no matter how off-the-cuff or jokingly said, may indicate serious suicidal feelings.

One of the most common misconceptions about talking with someone who might be contemplating suicide is that bringing up the subject may make things worse. This is not true. There is no danger of "giving someone the idea." Rather, the opposite is correct. Bringing up the question of suicide and discussing it without showing shock or disapproval is one of the most helpful things you can do. This openness shows that you are taking the individual seriously and responding to the severity of his or her distress.

If you do find that your friend or loved one is contemplating suicide, it is essential to help him or her find immediate professional care. (Calling the NAMI HelpLine at 1-800-950-NAMI [6264] for more information or to help you locate your local NAMI for area assistance is one possible resource.) Don't make the common misjudgment that those contemplating suicide are unwilling to seek help. Studies of suicide victims show that more than half had sought medical help within six months before their deaths. And don't leave the suicidal person to find help alone—they usually aren't capable. Also, never assume that someone who is determined to end his or her life can't be stopped. Even the most severely depressed person has mixed feelings about death, wavering until the very last moment between wanting to live and wanting to die. Most suicidal people do not want death; they want the pain to stop. The impulse to end it all, though, no matter how overpowering, does not last forever.

If the threat is immediate, if your friend or loved one tells you he or she is going to commit suicide, you must act immediately. Don't leave the person alone, and don't try to argue. Instead, ask questions like, "Have you thought about how you'd do it?" "Do you have the means?" and "Have you decided when you'll do it?" If the person has a defined plan, the means are easily available, the method is a lethal one, and the time is set, the risk of suicide is obviously severe. In such an instance, you must take the individual to the nearest psychiatric facility or hospital emergency room. If you are together on the phone, you may even need to call 911 or the police. Remember, under such circumstances no actions on your part should be considered too extreme—you are trying to save a life. An overwhelming majority of young people who hear a suicide threat from a friend or loved one don't report the threat to an adult. Take all threats seriously—you are not betraying someone's trust by trying to keep them alive.

Other Serious Considerations

Don't automatically assume that someone who was considering suicide and is now in treatment or tells you that he or she is feeling better is, in fact, doing better. Some who commit suicide actually do so just as they seem to be improving. One reason for this may be that they did not have enough energy to kill themselves when they were extremely depressed, but now have just enough energy to go through with their plan. Another reason for suicide during a seeming improvement is that resigning oneself to death can release

☞ Remember!!

Suicide is the third-leading cause of death for young people between the ages of 15 and 24 years. Behavioral indicators and threats of suicide should be taken seriously. Don't be afraid to report the threat to an adult. If you need more information, the resources on the next pages or at the end of this book may be helpful.

anxiety. While it's not good to monitor every action of someone who is recovering from suicidal thoughts, it is important to make certain that the lines of communication between you and the individual remain open.

While it may seem a bit obvious, it should also be mentioned that it is extremely advisable to bar teens who are suicidal from access to firearms. Nearly 60 percent of all completed suicides are committed with a firearm. And while having a firearm does not in itself promote suicidal behavior, knowing that one is accessible may help a troubled teen formulate his or her suicidal plans.

Support Groups And Organizations

American Academy of Child and Adolescent Psychiatry
3615 Wisconsin Avenue, N.W.
Washington, DC 20016
Phone: 202-966-7300
Fax: 202-966-2891
Website: http://www.aacap.org

American Association of Suicidology (AAS)
4201 Connecticut Avenue, N.W.
Suite 408
Washington, DC 20008
Phone: 202-237-2280
Fax: 202-237-2282
Website: http://www.suicidology.org

American Foundation for Suicide Prevention
120 Wall Street, 22nd Floor
New York, NY 10005
Toll Free: 888-333-AFSP
Phone: 212-363-3500
Fax: 212-363-6237
Website: http://www0.afsp.org/
E-Mail: inquiry@afsp.org

SPAN (Suicide Prevention Advocacy Network)
5034 Odin's Way
Marietta, GA 30068
Toll Free: 888-649-1366
Fax: 770-642-1419
Website: http://www.spanusa.org
E-Mail: act@spanusa.org

Suicide Awareness\Voices of Education (SA\VE)
P.O. Box 24507
Minneapolis, MN 55424-0507
Phone: 952-946-7998
Website: http://www.save.org
E-Mail: save@winternet.com

Suicide Information and Education Centre
#201 1615 10th Avenue, SW
Calgary, Alberta T3C 0J7
Phone: 403-245-3900
Fax: 403-245-0299
Website: http://www.siec.ca
E-Mail: siec@suicideinfo.ca

Yellow Ribbon Suicide Prevention Program
P.O. Box 644
Westminster, CO 80030-0644
Phone: 303-429-3530
Fax: 303-426-4496
Website: http://www.yellowribbon.org
E-Mail: ask4help@yellowribbon.org

Books

Jamison, Kay Redfield. *Night Falls Fast: Understanding Suicide*. Knopf, 1999.

Steel, Danielle. *His Bright Light: The Story of Nick Traina*. Delacorte Press, 1998.

Wrobleski, Adina. *Suicide: Why?* Afterwords, 1995.

Chapter 37

Depression And Substance Abuse Can Be A Lethal Combination

The teen years are a period of turmoil for just about everyone. Learning new social roles, developing new relationships, getting used to bodily changes, making decisions about the future—all of these things can be overwhelming. With neither the comforting dependence of childhood nor the full-fledged membership in adulthood, teens often feel as if they were floating in limbo—isolated, confused, scared, and alone.

It is not surprising then, that depression is a common illness among adolescents. The feelings of helplessness and hopelessness that accompany depression can fuel a downward spiral of health and self-esteem, which can have potentially deadly results: In one study of teenage suicides, 60 to 70 percent of the teens had been diagnosed with a depressive illness prior to their deaths. An alarming 90 percent of the sample had some form of psychiatric diagnosis—depression, mood disorder, or substance abuse disorder.

According to David Shaffer, M.D., adolescent depression often is complicated further by substance use problems. In one study, nearly 45 percent of the teens who had committed suicide in a two-year period, had been abusing alcohol at the time of their deaths.

About This Chapter: Text in this chapter is from " Depression and substance use can be a lethal combination for teens," in *The Addiction Letter*, June 1996, vol. 12, no. 6, p. S1(2), © Manisses Communications Group 1996; reprinted with permission.

What To Look For

Teens who are contemplating suicide often show symptoms of depression and/or substance use. The following symptoms typically indicate a problem:

- sleep disturbances—fatigue, frequent napping, early waking
- change in appetite—sudden noticeable weight loss or gain
- restlessness, inability to concentrate
- dramatic mood changes
- feelings of hopelessness, helplessness, despair
- withdrawal from friends and previously enjoyed activities

Teens who are depressed and abuse substances are at high risk for attempting suicide. If you think that your teen might be at risk, contact a professional immediately. Early intervention can prevent suicide attempts, and your teen can receive treatment for depression and for substance use.

> ♣ **It's A Fact!!**
>
> Alcohol and other drugs may temporarily ease the pain of depression, but they can also contribute to impulsive acts—like suicide.

Other Risk Factors

Young people who have attempted suicide in the past or who talk about suicide are at greater risk for future attempts. Listen for hints like, "I'd be better off dead," or "I won't be a problem for you much longer," or "Nothing matters; it's no use."

Adolescents who consider suicide generally feel alone, hopeless, and rejected. They are more vulnerable to having these feelings if they have been abused, feel that they have been humiliated recently in front of family or friends, or have chaotic, disorganized family lives.

Teenagers who are planning to commit suicide might "clean house" by giving away their favorite possessions, cleaning their rooms, or throwing things away. They also may become suddenly cheerful after a period of depression, because they think that they have found a solution by deciding to commit suicide.

One of the most dangerous times of a teen's life is when he or she has suffered a loss or humiliation of some kind—loss of self-esteem by doing poorly on an important test, breakup with a boyfriend or girlfriend, parents' divorce, for example.

What You Can Do

Most people who are depressed or who are thinking about suicide don't or won't talk about how they're feeling. They deny their emotions or think that talking about it will be a burden on others because no one cares. Or they are afraid other people will criticize or make fun of them.

If someone brings up the subject of suicide with you, take it seriously and take some time to talk about it. Reassure the person that he or she has someone to turn to. Remind the person of all the people who care about him or her—friends, family members, school counselors, physicians, or teachers.

Don't lecture or point out all the reasons the person has to live. Instead, listen and reassure him or her that the depression and suicidal tendencies can be treated.

Get help immediately. Don't wait for the symptoms to worsen. Contact the resources listed in this book, or check the yellow pages for the local chapter of the American Psychiatric Association. Don't attempt to solve the problem alone, and don't assume that the person is not serious.

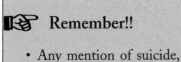 **Remember!!**

- Any mention of suicide, even in what appears to be jest, should be considered seriously.

- Teens who are contemplating suicide often show symptoms of depression and/or substance use.

- Early intervention can prevent suicide attempts.

Chapter 38

Thought Patterns That Predict Suicide Attempts

Suicidal Intent In Adolescents

For some adolescents, a suicide attempt is the result of impulsive behavior, typically in the face of significant stress. For others, a suicide attempt follows a course from passive suicidal ideation to serious consideration of suicide as an option, followed by active planning. For the latter group, the cognitive factors that contribute to suicidal behavior are particularly important to investigate.

The importance of an individual's cognitive constructs in understanding suicidal behavior is evident in various models that have been postulated regarding suicidal behavior. In our own model, and those developed by other research teams, pre-existing psychopathology, environmental factors and interpersonal problems are believed to affect thought processes and coping behaviors, which in turn lead to suicidal intent and behavior.

These cognitive factors, which include hopelessness, negative attributional style and problem solving, are believed to mediate the effects of these pre-existing factors or to have direct effects on suicidal intent and behavior.

About This Chapter: Text in this chapter is from "Cognitive characteristics predict adolescent suicide attempts," by Anthony Spirito in *The Brown University Child and Adolescent Behavior Letter*, June 1997, vol. 13, no. 6, p. 1(3), © 1997 Manisses Communications Group Inc.; reprinted with permission.

Cognitive processes at the time of the attempt are important to evaluate. In one of our studies, three primary aspects of suicide intent specific to adolescent suicide attempters emerged in a factor analysis of the Suicide Intent Scale. Two of the factors were primarily cognitive: they were labeled "expected outcome" and "planning activities," while the third we described as "isolation behaviors."

> ✎ **Weird Words**
>
> Cognition: Intellectual (rather than emotional) mental activities related to learning and thinking, including perception, reasoning, judgment, and memory.
>
> Psychopathology: The study of the nature or causes of mental diseases and behavior disorders.

"Expected outcome" refers to expectations, purpose, and perceived lethality of the suicide attempt. For example, in our study of almost 200 suicide attempters, about a third expected their suicide attempt would result in death. "Planning activities" include cognitions related to degree of premeditation and planning of the attempts.

Impulsive suicide attempts occurred in approximately two-thirds of the sample, while planned attempts were characteristic of about one-third of the group. We found that those adolescents who planned a suicide attempt were more hopeless and depressed and experienced significantly greater suicidal ideation than adolescents who made impulsive suicide attempts.

Hopelessness Versus Depression

Hopelessness has been discussed by many as a particularly important contributor to suicidal behavior. Hopelessness, which refers to a negative attitude about future events, including a global expectation of negative future occurrences, has been found to be consistently higher in suicide attempters than in suicide ideators, nonsuicidal psychiatrically hospitalized adolescents, and nonsuicidal adolescents in our studies. A number of studies, however, have shown that depression is more highly related to suicidal ideation than hopelessness, suggesting that hopelessness is more salient in attempters than in those who only think about it.

In one of our studies, hopelessness was more strongly related to suicide attempters than were other factors, including family dysfunction. Whether or not they are suicidal, female adolescents typically report higher levels of hopelessness than males.

Some adolescent suicide attempters also tend to have a negative attributional style; that is, they attribute undesirable events to themselves, to stable factors, and to global causes more often than nonsuicidal adolescents do.

However, in general, suicide attempters do not appear to be very different from nonsuicidal psychiatric patients in their attributional style. In one of our studies, suicide attempters were more likely than nonsuicidal psychiatric patients to attribute good events to global causes and negative events to stable aspects of their environment. This negative attributional style may help explain the cognitive set related to suicide attempts.

Five Steps To Problem SOLVEing

✤ It's A Fact!!

Surveys indicate that anywhere from 7 to 10 percent of adolescents report they have attempted suicide, and of these, approximately 2 to 3 percent receive medical care.

The other common cognitive factor studied in suicidal adolescents is problem-solving. Several studies have shown suicide attempters to have poorer interpersonal problem-solving ability than nonpsychiatrically distributed adolescents. In addition, adolescent suicide attempters report greater deficits in the problem-solving process than other groups when confronted with problematic situations. They have difficulty generating alternative solutions and identifying positive consequences for problem solutions, and they have limited flexibility that inhibits the problem solving process: These adolescents are not typically able to progress through the various steps needed to adequately solve a problem.

The acronym SOLVE can be used to describe these steps: Select problem, Options, Likely outcomes, Very best one to do, and Evaluate and repeat as necessary.

Overall, it appears that cognitive deficits, such as problem-solving and other cognitive distortions, appear in a significant portion of adolescent suicide attempters compared to nonsuicidal adolescents. It is unclear whether these are temporary deficits evident at the time of acute stress or more stable characteristics. One study suggests the deficits may be temporary: Psychiatrically hospitalized suicide attempters did not differ from controls in their overall ability to generate solutions to standardized personal problems, but they used fewer coping strategies than controls in response to their most recent severe stressor.

A lack of cognitive flexibility, assuming more responsibility for negative outcomes than may be necessary, and rigidity in problem solving, especially interpersonal problem solving, are evident in many adolescent suicide attempters seen in therapy.

Specific Treatment Interventions

As part of the initial assessment of an adolescent who has attempted suicide, the cognitive characteristics discussed above should be assessed via an interview or by using measures designed to tap these characteristics. Cognitive therapy techniques to address cognitive deficits, along with problem-solving therapy to help teach adolescents new ways of conceptualizing their problems and generating alternatives, should be considered whenever clinicians identify these cognitive deficits in adolescents seen following a suicide attempt. Monitoring thinking patterns in order to teach the relationship between cognitions and both emotions and behavior is often necessary.

Challenging the validity of negative thought patterns is a technique often used for suicidal adolescents. Other techniques include decatastrophizing; that is, helping adolescent suicide attempters re-evaluate whether they are

> ♣ It's A Fact!!
> Some suicides occur as a result of impulsive action. For others, a suicide attempt follows a course from passive suicidal ideation to serious consideration of suicide as an option, followed by active planning.

overestimating the catastrophic nature of their problems. By exploring various possibilities, the therapist helps the adolescent view the situation as difficult, but not impossible.

Another technique involves scaling the severity of events (for example, from 1 to 100) to prevent the adolescent from conceptualizing everything as black and white. A third technique is to have the adolescent make a list of actions that might be taken in response to the suicide precipitant and then rank the actions from least difficult to most difficult. A discussion regarding the least difficult choices then ensues. This helps move the adolescent away from thinking of suicide as the only option to thinking of it as the worst choice among several options.

The cognitive strategy that has been advocated most among clinicians working with adolescent suicide attempters is problem solving. In problem-solving therapy, the adolescent is taught new ways to conceptualize the problem, consider solutions and plan a course of action based on this information. By working with the adolescent to approach problems one at a time and generate alternative solutions, a therapist can help restore hope in what appears to be a hopeless situation.

About The Author

Anthony Spirito, PhD, is director of child psychology at Rhode Island Hospital in Providence, RI, sad associate professor of psychiatry at the Brown University School of Medicine. He has conducted clinical research with adolescent suicide attempters for the past 12 years.

Chapter 39

Questions Teens Often Ask About The Why And How Of Suicide

As a mental health practitioner, I have worked with teenagers for more than 30 years. For the past 14 years, since my family and I lost our 18-year-old son, Kevin, to suicide, I have been talking to teenagers about suicide, and more importantly, listening to their questions on the subject. Three questions come up repeatedly: WHY would someone want to kill himself or herself? WHAT can you do when you know a person who is suicidal and who won't let you help? And, HOW do people commit suicide?

Statistics show that since 1955, the teen suicide rate has risen nearly 400 percent. Between 1957 and 1987, the number of completed suicides rose 312 percent for youth between the ages of 15 and 19. And suicide deaths for children under age 15 are rising dramatically. Estimates indicate more than half of high-school students have thought about suicide.

In my years of addressing the subject, I've learned that the stigma surrounding suicide is so great that some teens hesitate to ask a question or make an observation in front of their peers. To counteract that dangerous hesitancy, I begin my presentations by telling of my experience with suicide,

About This Chapter: The text in this chapter is from "Teenagers commonly question the why and how of suicide," by Brian Barr in *The Brown University Child and Adolescent Behavior Letter*, December 1998, vol. 14, issue 12, p. 1, © 1998 Manisses Communications Group Inc.; reprinted with permission.

invite them write any questions they have about suicide on a three-by-five card and return it to me anonymously. I assure them that if I haven't answered their question in the course of my presentation, I will look at each card and answer all questions before I conclude.

Teens respond positively to both the privacy afforded in writing out questions and the assurance that, before our time together ends, their questions will be answered. This is particularly meaningful when addressing a series of classes or groups. Word spreads fast, and when you honor your commitment to answer questions in one group, the groups that follow feel confident that they, too, will be answered.

Why?

The leading question by far is always why. Why would someone want to kill himself or herself? I answer by emphasizing the well-known risk factors such as previous attempts, substance abuse, mental health problems, issues surrounding sexual orientation and, especially, depression. Most teenagers are not aware that if they experience depression and let it go untreated, it is an inherent threat to their well-being. They have little awareness of the danger untreated depression can have to their family, social and personal relationships as well as to their academic and other critical adjustments. It is important to tell them that the pain that comes with depression can be so intolerable that a person will do whatever they can to escape it.

The preventive message: If ever you dwell upon the thought that the world would be a better place without you, you must seek help immediately.

How Can You Help Someone Who Is Suicidal?

The second most frequently asked question is, "What can you do about a person you know who is suicidal and who won't let you help?"

This question inevitably is asked in writing by very concerned teens. My regard for our young people is greatly reaffirmed because they have such inherent decency and concern for one another.

This question more than any other provides an opportunity to relieve a tired and frustrated teen of an enormous burden. Once they know, as do our professionals, that when someone is experiencing serious depression that person may be unable to accept normal reaching out and, in fact, may push away a well-meaning friend, it gives them the understanding they need to make a significant difference for the person at risk.

Teens are amazingly relieved to learn that their felt rejection is a symptom of the other person's distress, and not a personal affront. After recognizing this, teens often tell me they are willing to stay the course, continue friendly dialogue and talk with a trusted adult about the situation. Knowledge does translate into action.

How Do People Commit Suicide?

Every reported survey shows suicide to be in the top three areas of concern expressed by teens. They spend a lot of time talking about it. Most of them know someone who died from suicide. Many have been thinking about it as an option and, regrettably, the Gallup surveys of 1991 and 1994 found that 6 percent have attempted suicide. It isn't that big a leap to understand their curiosity about the "how" of terminating life.

When this question is asked, I always discuss the lethality of guns and the fact that more than 60 percent of completed suicides result from a self-inflicted gunshot. In a household where someone has talked of suicide, or demonstrated any other signs that he or she might be thinking of taking his or her life, access to such deadly weapons must be totally restricted.

There are always other questions, of course, but these three continue to be the most often asked. Anytime a question is asked about suicide, we are given a unique opportunity to bring light, and ultimately power, to our young people, who can convert the knowledge and energy into self-protection.

References

If you have additional questions about suicide and suicide prevention, these resources provide more in-depth information. Ask your school or public librarian for assistance in locating the documents that interest you.

Zenere FJ, Lazarus PJ: The decline of youth suicidal behavior in an urban, multicultural public school system following the introduction of a suicide prevention and intervention. *Suicide and Life-Threatening Behavior* 1997; 27(4):387-403.

Maris RW, Silverman MM: Postscript: Summary and synthesis. *Suicide and Life Threatening Behavior* 1995; 25(1):205-209.

Pataki CS, Carlson GA: Childhood and adolescent depression: A review. *Harvard Rev Psychiatry* 1995; 3(1): 140-151.

Gallup Organization. *Teen Suicide Study*. Insurance Research Group. 1991.

Gallup Organization. *Teen Suicide Study*. Insurance Research Group. 1994.

Centers for Disease Control and Prevention (CDC). *Youth suicide prevention programs: A resource guide*. Atlanta: U.S. Department of Health and Human Services, Public Health Service, CDC, 1992.

—by Brian Barr, C.S.W., C.A.S.A.C.

W. Brian Barr is a certified social worker and a credentialed alcoholism and drug abuse counselor. He is associate commissioner of the State of New York Office of Children and Family Services.

Chapter 40

Fifteen Myths About Teen Suicide

Adolescent suicide represents the second leading cause of death among 15-19 year olds.[1] In 1994, 2,270 youth died from suicide.[2] Considering that medical examiners underreport suicides by 25% to 50%,[3] and that 100 to 200 suicide attempts occur per youth suicide completion,[2] 1994 may actually have experienced as many as 4,500 youth suicides and 900,000 youth suicide attempts.

Fortunately, increasing attention to this issue is occurring, and school suicide prevention programs are being implemented throughout the United States. Unfortunately, many myths persist regarding adolescent suicide. Such myths could undercut the effectiveness of suicide prevention programs. This chapter addresses 15 prevalent myths about adolescent suicide and the facts that correspond to each.

Fifteen Prevalent Myths

Myth 1. Adolescent suicide is a decreasing problem in the United States.

While the suicide rate for the general population has remained relatively stable since the 1950s, the suicide rate for adolescents has more than tripled.[2]

About This Chapter: Text in this chapter is from "Fifteen Prevalent Myths Concerning Adolescent Suicide," by Keith A. King, *Journal of School Health*, April 1999, vol. 69, issue 4, p. 159, © 1999 American School Health Association. Reprinted with permission. American School Health Association, Kent, Ohio.

♣ **It's A Fact!!**

Many internet sites can give you additional information about teen suicide.

American Foundation for Suicide Prevention
Web site: www.afsp.org

Provides research, education, and current statistics regarding suicide. Links to other suicide and mental health sites are offered. Membership opportunity available.

Suicide Awareness\Voices of Education
Web site: www.save.org

Provides suicide education, facts, and statistics on suicide and suicide and depression. Links to information on warning signs of suicide and the role a friend or family member can play in helping a suicidal person. Information can be sent via e-mail.

Suicide@rochford.org
Web site: www.rochford.org/suicide

Information about warning signs, answers to frequently asked questions, current statistics, and interactive features are provided.

American Association of Suicidology
Web site: www.suicidology.org

Resource for anyone concerned about suicide. Provides information on current research, prevention, ways to help a suicidal person, and surviving suicide. A list of crisis centers is also included.

Australian Institute for Suicide Research and Prevention
Web site: www.gu.edu.au/school/psy/aisrap

Provides information on youth suicide, suicide and families, and guidelines for the role of a helper.

Youth—Depression and Suicide
Web site: www.jaring.my/befrienders/youth1.htm

Offers information on warning signs and ways to help suicidal and depressed youth.

Presently, the suicide rate for 15-24 year-olds stands at 13.8 per 100,000.[2] From 1980 to 1992, the suicide rate for 15-19 year-olds and 10-14 year-olds increased 28% and 120%, respectively.[4]

Myth 2. Adolescent homicide is more common than adolescent suicide.

For adolescents 15-19 years of age, suicide is the second leading cause of death, and homicide is the third leading cause of death.[2] For adults, suicide is also more common than homicide. In US adults, suicide is presently the ninth leading cause of death and homicide is the 10th leading cause of death.[2]

Myth 3. Most adolescent suicides occur unexpectedly without warning signs.

Nine of 10 adolescents who commit suicide give clues to others before the suicide attempt.[5] Warning signs for adolescent suicide include depressed mood, substance abuse, loss of interest in once-pleasurable activities, decreased activity levels, decreased attention, distractability, isolation, withdrawing from others, sleep changes, appetite changes, morbid ideation, offering verbal cues ("I wish I were dead"), offering written cues (notes, poems), and giving possessions away.[6,7]

In addition, the following risk factors place an adolescent at increased risk for suicidal behavior: having a previous suicide attempt, having a recent relationship breakup, being impulsive, having low self-esteem, being homosexual, coming from an abusive home, having easy access to a firearm, having low grades, and being exposed to suicide or suicidal behavior by another person.[6,8-10] Moreover, most suicidal adolescents attempt to communicate their suicidal thoughts to another in some manner.[11] Not surprisingly, an effective way to prevent adolescent suicide involves learning to identify the warning signs of someone at risk.[7]

Myth 4. Adolescents who talk about suicide do not attempt or commit suicide.

One of the most ominous warning signs of adolescent suicide involves talking repeatedly about one's own death.[10,12] Adolescents who make threats of suicide should be taken seriously and provided the help that they need.[6] In this manner suicide attempts can be averted and lives can be saved.

Myth 5. Most adolescents who attempt suicide fully intend to die.

Most suicidal adolescents do not want suicide to happen.[13] Rather, they feel torn between wanting to end their psychological pain through death and wanting to continue living, though only in a more hopeful environment. Such ambivalence is communicated to others through verbal statements and behavior changes in 80% of suicidal youth.[7]

Myth 6. Educating teens about suicide leads to increased suicide attempts, since it provides them with ideas and methods about killing themselves.

When issues concerning suicide are taught in a sensitive context, education does not lead to, or cause, further suicidal behavior.[14] Since three-fourths (77%) of teen-age students state that if they were contemplating suicide they would first turn to a friend for help,[15] peer assistance programs have been implemented throughout the nation. Educational programs help students identify peers at risk and help them receive the help they need. Such programs have been associated with increased student knowledge about suicide warning signs and how to contact a hotline or crisis center, as well as increased likelihood to refer other students at risk to school counselors and mental health professionals.[16] Further, directly asking adolescents if they are thinking about suicide displays care and concern and may help in clearly determining whether or not an adolescent is considering suicide.[6,11]

Myth 7. Adolescents cannot relate to a person who has experienced suicidal thoughts.

Data from the 1997 *Youth Risk Behavior Surveillance Survey (YRBS)*,[17] which surveyed 16,262 high school students, found that one in five students (24.1%) had seriously considered attempting suicide in the previous year. A population study of 5,000 teen-agers from a rural community showed that 40% had entertained ideas of suicide at some point in their lives.[18] Some researchers estimated that it is more realistic that more than one-half of all high school students have experienced thoughts of suicide.[19] Further, a Midwestern survey of more than 400 junior and senior high school students found that almost one-half of the students reported knowing a friend who had attempted suicide.[20]

Myth 8. No difference exists between male and female adolescents regarding suicidal behavior.

Adolescent females are significantly more likely than adolescent males to have thought about suicide and to have attempted suicide.[17] Specifically, adolescent females are 1.5 to 2 times more likely than adolescent males to report experiencing suicidal ideation and 3 to 4 times more likely to attempt suicide.[9,17] Adolescent males are 4 to 5.5 times more likely than adolescent females to complete a suicide attempt.[9,21] While adolescent females complete one of every 25 suicide attempts, adolescent males complete one of every three attempts.[20]

Myth 9. Because female adolescents complete suicide at a lower rate than male adolescents, their attempts should not be taken too seriously.

One of the most powerful predictors of completed suicide is a prior suicide attempt.[10] Adolescents who attempted suicide are eight times more likely than adolescents who have not attempted suicide to attempt suicide again.[22] One-third to one-half of adolescents who kill themselves have a history of a previous suicide attempt.[23,24] Therefore, all suicide attempts should be treated seriously, regardless of gender.

Myth 10. The most common method for adolescent suicide completion involves drug overdose.

Guns are the most frequently used method for completing suicides among adolescents.[25] In 1994, guns accounted for 67% of all completed adolescent suicides, while strangulation (by hanging), the second most frequently used method for adolescent suicide completions, accounted for 18% of all completed adolescent suicides.[30] A gun in the house increases an adolescent's risk of suicide. Regardless of whether a gun is locked up or not, its presence in the home is associated with a higher risk for adolescent suicide,[26] even after controlling for most psychiatric variables. Homes with guns are 4.8 times more likely to experience a suicide of a resident than homes without guns.[27] Thus, it should not be surprising that restricting access to handguns significantly decreases suicide rates among 15-24 year-olds.[28,29]

Myth 11. All adolescents who engage in suicidal behavior are mentally ill.

Most adolescents have entertained thoughts about suicide at least once in their lives. Though there are some cases of adolescents attempting and completing suicide as a result of a mental disorder, most are not suffering from a mental disorder.[6] Studies involving psychological autopsies of adolescents who completed suicide suggest most adolescents are relatively rational and coherent at the time of their death.[6]

Myth 12. If adolescents want to commit suicide, there is nothing anyone can do to prevent its occurrence.

One of the most important things an individual can do to prevent suicide is to identify the warning signs of suicide and recognize an adolescent at increased risk for suicide.[30] School professionals should be aware of these risk factors and know how to respond when a student threatens or attempts suicide.[19] The existence of a school crisis intervention team may assist with this process.

Myth 13. Suicidal behavior is inherited.

No specific suicide gene has been identified.[7] Studies involving twins found higher concordance rates for suicide in monozygotic twins than in dizygotic twins, meaning that an identical twin would be more likely than a fraternal twin to engage in suicidal behavior if the co-twin committed suicide.[31] However, no study to date has examined the concordance for suicide in monozygotic twins separated at birth and raised apart, a requirement necessary to be met as a means to indicate inheritance of psychiatric illness.[7] Such a study could assess the effects that parental rearing style and familial environment have on suicidal behavior. When compared to control subjects, adolescent suicide victims have significantly less-frequent and less-satisfying communication with their parents.[32]

Myth 14. Adolescent suicide occurs only among poor adolescents.

Adolescent suicide occurs in all socioeconomic groups.[5,7] Socioeconomic variables have not proven reliable predictors of adolescent suicidal behavior.[7] Instead of assessing adolescents' socioeconomic backgrounds, school professionals should assess their social and emotional characteristics such as affect, mood, and social involvement to determine if they are at increased risk.

Myth 15. Only a counselor or a mental health professional can help a suicidal adolescent.

Most adolescents contemplating suicide are not seeing a mental health professional.[14] Rather, most are likely to approach a family member, peer, or school professional for help.[33-35] Displaying concern and care as well as ensuring that the adolescent is referred to a mental health professional are ways paraprofessionals can help.[12,14]

☞ Remember!!

In attempting to reduce suicide among adolescents, school professionals must possess accurate information. Remaining aware of and refuting the myths of adolescent suicide will assist in this process. All school staff must feel they have a responsibility to play in preventing suicide for an effective and comprehensive suicide prevention program to take effect.

References

1. Berman AL, Jobes DA. Suicide prevention in adolescents (age 12-18). *Suicide Life-Threaten Behav.* 1995;25:143-154.

2. National Center for Health Statistics. Advance report of final mortality statistics, 1994. *NCHS Monthly Vital Statistics Report.* 1996;45(suppl.3).

3. Jobes DA, Casey JO, Berman AL, Wright DG. Empirical criteria for the determination of suicide manner of death. *J Forensic Sci.* 1991;36:244-256.

4. Centers for Disease Control. Suicide among children, adolescents, and young adults—United States, 1980-1992. *MMWR.* 1995;44(15):290-291.

5. Curran DF. *Adolescent Suicidal Behavior.* Washington, DC: Hemisphere Publishing; 1987.

6. Kirk WG. *Adolescent Suicide. A School-based Approach to Assessment and Intervention.* Champaign, Ill: Research Press; 1993.

7. Lester DL. *Making Sense of Suicide: An In-depth Look at Why People Kill Themselves.* Philadelphia, Pa: The Charles Press Publishers, Inc; 1997.

8. Brent DA, Perper JA, Mortiz G, et al. Psychiatric risk factors for adolescent suicide: a case-controlled study. *J Am Acad Child Adolesc Psychiatry.* 1993;32:521-529.

9. King CA. Suicidal behavior in adolescence. In: Maris RW, Silverman MM, Canetto CA, eds. *Review of Suicidology, 1997.* New York, NY: The Guilford Press; 1997.

10. Committee on Adolescence. Group for the Advancement of Psychiatry. *Adolescent Suicide.* Washington, DC: American Psychiatric Press, Inc; 1996.

11. Hicks BB. *Youth Suicide: A Comprehensive Manual for Prevention and Intervention.* Bloomington, Ind: National Education Service; 1990.

12. Hoff LA. Crisis intervention in schools. In: Leenaars AA, Wenckstern S, eds. *Suicide Prevention in Schools.* New York, NY: Hemisphere Publishing Corp; 1991.

13. Smith J. Suicide intervention in schools: General considerations. In: Leenaars AA, Wenckstern S, eds. *Suicide Prevention in Schools.* New York, NY: Hemisphere Publishing Corp; 1991.

14. Tierney R, Ramsay R, Tanney B, Lang W. Comprehensive school suicide prevention programs. In: Leenaars AA, Wenckstern S, eds. *Suicide Prevention in Schools.* New York, NY: Hemisphere Publishing Corp; 1991.

15. Gallup G. *The Gallup Survey on Teenage Suicide*. Princeton, NJ: The George H. Gallup International Institute; 1991.

16. McEvoy M, LeClaire D. The PAL (Peer Assistant Leadership) program: a comprehensive model for suicide prevention. Presented at conference of the National Organization of Student Assistance Programs and Partners; 1993; Chicago, Ill.

17. Centers for Disease Control. Youth risk behavior surveillance—United States, 1997. *MMWR*. 1998;47(SS-3):1-89.

18. Whitaker A, Shaffer D. Suicidal ideation in a non-referred adolescent population. Presented at the Roddy Brickell Symposium at the New York State Psychiatric Institute; March 16, 1993.

19. McKee PW, Jones RW, Barbe RH. *Suicide and the School: A Practical Guide to Suicide Prevention*. Horsham, Pa: LRP Publications; 1993.

20. Karolus S, Kirk WG, Shatz M. Identification of suicidal symptoms by high school students. Presented at annual meeting of the Illinois School Psychologists Association; February 1990; Champaign, Ill.

21. National Center for Health Statistics. *National Vital Statistics Report*. 1998;47(suppl 9).

22. Lewinsohn P, Rohde P, Seeley JR. Psychosocial characteristics of adolescents with a history of suicide attempt. *J Am Soc Child Adoles Health Care*. 1993;4:106-108.

23. Hawton K, Catalan J. *Attempted Suicide: A Practical Guide to its Nature and Management*. Oxford: Oxford University Press; 1987.

24. Marttunen MJ, Aro HM, Lonnqvist JK. Adolescence and suicide: a review of psychological autopsy studies. *Eur Child Adolesc Psychiatry*. 1993;2:10-18.

25. Marttunen M J, Aro HM, Lonnqvist JK. Adolescent suicide: endpoint of long-term difficulties. *J Am Acad Child Adolesc Psychiatry*. 1992;31:649-654.

26. Brent DA, Perper JA, Allman C J, Moritz GM, Wartella ME, Zellenak JP. The presence and accessibility of firearms in the homes of adolescent suicides: a case-controlled study. *JAMA*. 1991;266:2989-2995.

27. Kellerman AL, Rivera FP, Somes G, et al. Suicide in the home in relationship to gun ownership. *N Engl J Med*. 1992;327:467-472.

28. Carrington PJ, Moyer S. Gun control and suicide in Ontario. *Am J Psychiatry*. 1994; 151:606-608.

29. Sloan JH, Rivera FP, Reay DT, et al. Firearms regulation and the rates of suicide: a comparison of two metropolitan areas. *N Engl J Med*. 1990;322:369-373.

30. Centers for Disease Control. Programs for the prevention of suicide among adolescent and young adults. Suicide contagion and the reporting of suicide. Recommendations from a national workshop. *MMWR*. 1994;43(RR6).

31. Lester D. Genetics, twin studies, and suicide. *Suicide Life-Threaten Behav*. 1986; 16:274-295.

32. Gould MS, Fisher P, Parides M, Flory M, Shaffer D. Psychosocial risk factors of child and adolescent completed suicide. *Arch Gen Psychiatry*. 1996;53:1155-1162.

33. Boldero J, Fallon B. Adolescent help-seeking: What do they get help for and from whom? *J Adolesc*. 1995;18:193-209.

34. Robins PR, Tanck RH. University students' preferred choices for social support. *J Soc Psychol*. 1995; 135:775-776.

35. Armacost RL. High school student stress and the role of counselors. *Sch Counselor*. 1990;38:105-112.

About The Author

Keith A. King, PhD, is Assistant Professor, Health Promotion, Health Promotion and Education Program, at the University of Cincinnati, Cincinnati, OH 45221-0002.

Chapter 41

If You Are Feeling Suicidal

If you are feeling suicidal, please contact your local crisis line or counseling center. There are several ways to find assistance:

By Phone

- Check your phone directory for the listing of your local crisis center.

- National Crisis Helpline—For use in locating the nearest crisis service in the United States: 1-800-999-9999

On Line Resources

- To access lists of Canadian and American crisis centers from the Suicide Information and Education Centre's web page go to **http:// www.siec.ca** and click on the SIEC box; then click on "If you are suicidal or concerned about someone."

- To find a crisis center in the United States, go to **http:// www.suicidology.org/index.html** and click on "Crisis Centers"

- To find a crisis center in Canada, go to **http://www.suicideinfo.ca/ support/canada/index.htm**

About This Chapter: Information in this chapter is from "If You Are Feeling Suicidal," produced by the Suicide Information and Education Centre (SIEC); © SIEC; reprinted with permission from SIEC. Website addresses and instructions updated in May 2001.

- To find a crisis hotline in the United States, Canada, or anywhere else in the world, go to **http://www.befrienders.org/bidir/centre.htm**

- On-line counseling is available at **http://www.befrienders.org/email.html** (This is a 24-hour confidential e-mail service provided by the Samaritans.)

- Special information and help for young people is available at **http://kidshelp.sympatico.ca** (This service also addresses issues other than suicide. For suicide information click on "Tools for Life" and then click on "Suicide.")

- If you are feeling suicidal, go to **http://www.metanoia.org/suicide** (This page contains conversations and writings for suicidal persons to read. If you're feeling at all suicidal, be sure to read this page before you take any action. It might just save your life.)

You have made the right choice to look for help. We hope you will contact someone right away.

If You Are Concerned About Someone

The Suicide Information and Education Centre (SIEC) is a library and resource center. If you use these SIEC guidelines, you are responsible for ensuring that they are appropriate to your needs and that you use them as intended. It is strongly recommended that you continue to seek assistance from a professional caregiver.

If you are concerned that someone you know may be thinking of suicide, you can help. Remember, as a helper, do not promise to do anything you do not want to do or that you cannot do.

First Of All

If the person is actively suicidal, get help immediately. Call your local crisis service or the police, or take the person to the emergency room of your local hospital. Do not leave the person alone.

If the person has attempted suicide and needs medical attention, call 9-1-1 or your local emergency services number.

Helping

The following are suggestions for helping someone who is suicidal:

- Ask the person: "Are you thinking of suicide?" Ask them if they have a plan and if they have the means. Asking someone if they are suicidal will not make them suicidal. Most likely they will be relieved that you have asked. Experts believe that most people are ambivalent about their wish to die.

- Listen actively to what the person is saying to you. Remain calm and do not judge what you are being told. Do not advise the person not to feel the way they are.

- Reassure the person that there is help for their problems and reassure them that they are not "bad" or "stupid" because they are thinking about suicide.

- Help the person break down their problem(s) into more manageable pieces. It is easier to deal with one problem at a time.

- Emphasize that there are ways other than suicide to solve problems. Help the person to explore these options, for example, ask them what else they could do to change their situation.

- Offer to investigate counseling services.

- Do not agree to keep the person's suicidal thoughts or plans a secret. Helping someone who is suicidal can be very stressful. Get help—ask family members and friends for their assistance and to share the responsibility.

- Suggest that the person see a doctor for a complete physical. Although there are many things that family and friends can do to help, there may be underlying medical problems that require professional intervention. Your doctor can also refer patients to a psychiatrist, if necessary.

- Try to get the person to see a trained counselor. Do not be surprised if the person refuses to go to a counselor—but be persistent. There are many types of caregivers for the suicidal. If the person will not go to a psychologist, or a psychiatrist, suggest, for example, they talk to a clergyperson, a guidance counselor, or a teacher.

We hope these suggestions will help you. Don't forget to check your phone directory for the number of the local crisis service. You can also access a list of crisis centers in Canada and the USA from the SIEC website at www.siec.ca.

☞ Remember!!

If you would like to talk to someone via the Internet, the Samaritans offer a confidential service at: http://www.befrienders.org/email.html

If you would like the Suicide Information and Education Centre to send you some resources on suicide prevention or suicide bereavement, you can e-mail SIEC at: siec@suicideinfo.ca. Please remember to include your mailing address—they cannot send these materials over the Internet. You can also contact SIEC at:

Suicide Information and Education Centre
#201 1615 10th Avenue, SW
Calgary, Alberta T3C 0J7
Phone: 403-245-3900
Fax: 403-245-0299
Website: http://www.siec.ca

Chapter 42

How To Prevent Suicide

It is a myth that suicide can't be prevented. It can. QPR is one technique that can help. QPR stands for "Question," "Persuade," and "Refer." Much like CPR or the Heimlich maneuver, the fundamentals of QPR are easily learned. And like CPR and the Heimlich maneuver, the application of QPR may save a life. The more people who are trained in this technique, the more lives that will be saved.

Research shows that the great majority of those who attempt suicide give some signal first. Yet those in a position to do something about it are often reluctant to get involved. Sometimes, because the thought of death is frightening, we deny the person may be suicidal. Overcoming the denial is an important step.

People who are thinking about suicide, are not necessarily being irrational. They look at it as a solution to their problems. What we have to do is make them realize there are other solutions.

Before applying QPR, you have to recognize the warning signs of suicide.

About This Chapter: Text in this chapter is paraphrased from "QPR, Ask a Question, Save a Life," by Paul Quinnett, Ph.D. To have this workshop presented to your organization, call 509-458-7171 or 1-800-256-6996. © National Alliance for the Mentally Ill (NAMI). Reprinted with permission of the National Alliance for the Mentally Ill. This information is a public service provided for educational purposes. Do not rely on it. Consult your doctor before making any decisions.

Direct Verbal Clues

- "I've decided to kill myself"
- "I wish I were dead"
- "I'm going to commit suicide"
- "If such and such doesn't happen, I'll kill myself"

Indirect Or Coded Verbal Cues

- "I'm tired of life"
- "What's the point of going on"
- "My family would be better off without me"
- "Who cares if I'm dead"
- "I can't go on anymore"
- "I just want out"
- "You would be better off without me"
- "Nobody needs me anymore"

Behavioral Clues

- Donating body to medical school
- Buying a gun
- Stockpiling pills
- Putting business affairs in order
- Changing a will

Situational Clues

- Sudden rejection or unexpected separation
- Death of someone close (especially by suicide)
- Diagnosis of terminal illness
- Anticipated loss of financial security or personal freedom

Sudden Happiness

- Sudden happiness in a depressed person may be signal of suicide.

Wishing to be dead is a frequent symptom of untreated depression. Since depression saps energy and purpose, sometimes the depressed person is 'too tired' to carry out a suicide plan. However, as the depression finally begins to lift, the person may suddenly feel 'well enough' to act. As strange as it sounds, once someone decides to end his or her suffering by suicide, the hours before death are often filled with a blissful calm. This sudden change in appearance is a good time to apply QPR.

What To Do

If someone is contemplating suicide, keep them sober.

People who take their lives have to pass a psychological barrier before they act. This final wall of resistance is what keeps many seriously suicidal people alive. Alcohol dissolves this wall and is found in the blood of most completed suicides. If someone is contemplating suicide, keep them sober.

Prevention Steps

The first step to preventing suicide is to **QUESTION**.

Get the person alone or in a private setting and ask the person if they are contemplating suicide. A crowded restaurant is a bad place to do this. Your own home may be a good one. Ask questions that acknowledge the individuals distress. Questions like, "Have you been unhappy lately?" "Do you ever wish you could go to sleep and not wake up?" Or you can ask directly, "Do you want to stop living?"

Asking the suicide question does not increase risk.

Giving a 'yes' answer to these questions is often a release for the individual. It makes them feel better, not worse. The suicide question is now on the table for discussion. But that also means you have obligations you did not have a minute ago.

After asking the question, you have to listen. Listen for the problems death by suicide would solve. Listening is the greatest gift one human can give to another. Advice tends to be easy, quick, cheap, and wrong. Listening takes time, patience, courage, but is always right. Give your full attention and don't interrupt. Do not judge or condemn. Listen for the problems death by suicide would solve.

The second step is to **PERSUADE** the individual to get help.

The goal of persuasion is to get the person to say 'yes', they will get help. Ask the following questions: "Will you go with me to see a counselor (priest, minister, nurse, etc.)?" "Will you let me help you make an appointment with....", "Will you promise me...."

Sometimes people will agree to get help and not get it or resist the idea of getting help. So you may want to make a "no-suicide" contract: a promise not to hurt oneself until help is gotten." Because making a promise appeals to our honor, and agreeing to stay safe relieves our suffering, the answer is almost always, yes.

If the answer is 'no', the individual is probably a "danger to self or others' and can (should) be involuntarily committed so they can access professional help. Call 911.

- Remind the person that there are better alternatives than suicide.
- Focus on other solutions to problems, not the suicide solution.
- Accept the reality of the person's pain and offer alternatives.
- Offer hope in any form and in any way.

Remove firearms, car keys, medications, knives, and other instruments which may be used to commit suicide. By restricting access to the means of suicide you buy time for another solution to be found. Removing the means to suicide is, in itself, an act of hope.

The final step in QPR is to make a **REFERRAL**.

Get the person to get help. NAMI is one source of referrals (call 800-950-NAMI). Go with them. The best referrals are when you personally take the person you are worried about to provider or appropriate professionals. If you are making a referral, don't worry about being disloyal, you are trying to save a life. Don't worry about breaking a trust or not having enough information to call for help. This gets in the way of helping.

Part 4

Getting Treatment

Chapter 43

Guidelines For Seeking Mental Health Care

Finding The Right Mental Health Care

If you or someone you know may benefit from a counselor or mental health center, here are some questions and guidelines to help you find the right care.

Where Do You Go For Help?

Where you go for help will depend on who has the problem (an adult or child) and the nature of the problem and/or symptoms. Often, the best place to start is your local Mental Health Association. Check your Yellow Pages for a listing or call the National Mental Health Association at 800-969-NMHA (6642).

Other suggested resources include:

• Your local health department's Mental Health Division. These services are state funded and are obligated to first serve individuals who meet "priority population criteria" for children and adults as defined by the state Mental Health Department. There may be waiting lists and not all individuals may be eligible for services.

About This Chapter: Text in this chapter is from "Mental Illness in the Family: Part 2—Guidelines for Seeking Care," publication #238 produced by the National Mental Health Association (NMHA); © 1997 NMHA. Reprinted with permission from the National Mental Health Association (1-800-969-NHMA).

- Other mental health organizations (see the chapter titled "Mental Health Resources" at the end of this book)
- Family physician
- Clergyperson
- Family services agencies, such as associated Catholic Charities, Family and Children's Services, or Jewish Social Services
- Educational consultants or school counselors
- Marriage and family counselors
- Child guidance counselors
- Psychiatric hospitals accredited by the joint Commission on Accreditation of Health Care Organizations
- Hotlines, crisis centers, and emergency rooms (call 411 for Directory Assistance)

Which Mental Health Professional Is Right For You?

There are many types of mental health professionals. Finding the right one for you may require some research. Often it is a good idea to first describe the symptoms and/or problems to your family physician or clergy. He or she may be able to suggest what type of mental health professional you should call.

Types Of Mental Health Professionals

Psychiatrist: Medical doctor with special training in the diagnosis and treatment of mental and emotional illnesses. Like other doctors, psychiatrists are qualified to prescribe medication.

Qualifications: A state license and be board eligible or certified by the American Board of Psychiatry and Neurology.

Child/Adolescent Psychiatrist: Medical doctor with special training in the diagnosis and treatment of emotional and behavioral problems in children. Child/Adolescent psychiatrists are qualified to prescribe medication.

Qualifications: A state license and be board eligible or certified by the American Board of Psychiatry and Neurology.

Psychologist: Counselor with an advanced degree from an accredited graduate program in psychology and 2 or more years of supervised work experience. Trained to make diagnoses and provide individual and group therapy.

Qualifications: A state license.

Clinical Social Worker: Counselor with a masters degree in social work from an accredited graduate program. Trained to make diagnoses and provide individual and group counseling.

Qualifications: State license; may be member of the Academy of Certified Social Workers.

Licensed Professional Counselor: Counselor with a masters degree in psychology, counseling, or a related field. Trained to diagnose and provide individual and group counseling.

Qualifications: A state license.

Mental Health Counselor: Counselor with a masters degree and several years of supervised clinical work experience. Trained to diagnose and provide individual and group counseling.

Qualifications: Certification by the National Academy of Certified Clinical Mental Health Counselors.

Certified Alcohol and Drug Abuse Counselor: Counselor with specific clinical training in alcohol and drug abuse. Trained to diagnose and provide individual and group counseling.

Qualifications: A state license.

Nurse Psychotherapist: A registered nurse who is trained in the practice of psychiatric and mental health nursing. Trained to diagnose and provide individual and group counseling.

Qualifications: Certification, a state license.

Marital and Family Therapist: A counselor with a masters degree, with special education and training in marital and family therapy. Trained to diagnose and provide individual and group counseling.

Qualifications: A state license.

♣ It's A Fact!!
Types Of Therapy

Psychotherapy is a method of talking face-to-face with a therapist. The following are a few of the types of available therapy:

Behavioral Therapy: Includes stress management, biofeedback, and relaxation training to change thinking patterns and behavior.

Psychoanalysis: Long-term therapy meant to "uncover" unconscious motivations and early patterns to resolve issues and to become aware of how those motivations influence present actions and feelings.

Cognitive Therapy: Seeks to identify and correct thinking patterns that can lead to troublesome feelings and behavior.

Family Therapy: Includes discussion and problem-solving sessions with every member of the family.

Movement/Art/Music Therapy: These methods include the use of movement, art, or music to express emotions. Effective for persons who cannot otherwise express feelings.

Group Therapy: Includes a small group of people who, with the guidance of a trained therapist, discuss individual issues and help each other with problems.

Medications: Drugs can be beneficial to some persons with mental or emotional disorders. The patient should ask about risk, possible side-effects, and interaction with certain foods, alcohol, and other medications. Medication should be taken in the prescribed dosage and at prescribed intervals and should be monitored daily.

Electroconvulsive Therapy (ECT): Used to treat some cases of major depression, delusions, and hallucinations, or life-threatening sleep and eating disorders that can not be effectively treated with drugs and/or psychotherapy. Discuss with your physician the risks and side effects of ECT.

Pastoral Counselor: Clergy with training in clinical pastoral education. Trained to diagnose and provide individual and group counseling.

Qualifications: Certification from American Association of Pastoral Counselors.

Choosing A Mental Health Professional

You made the call to the mental health professional, now what do you do? Ask about his or her style and philosophy of working with patients, whether or not he or she has a specialty or concentration (some psychologists for instance specialize in family counseling, or child counseling, while others specialize in divorce or coping with the loss of a loved one). If you feel comfortable talking to the counselor or doctor, the next step is to make an appointment.

On your first visit, the counselor or the doctor, will want to get to know you and why you called him or her. The counselor will want to know: what you think the problem is, about your life, what you do, where you live, with whom you live. It is also common to be asked about your family and friends. This information helps the professional to assess your situation and develop a plan for treatment.

If you don't feel comfortable with the professional after the first, or even several visits, talk about your feelings at your next meeting. Don't be afraid to contact another counselor. Feeling comfortable with the professional you choose is very important to the success of your treatment.

What About Self-Help/Support Groups?

Self-help support groups bring together people with common experiences. Participants share experiences, provide understanding and support and help each other find new ways to cope with problems.

There are support groups for almost any concern including alcoholism, overeating, the loss of a child, co-dependency, grandparenting, various mental illnesses, cancer, parenting, and many, many others.

✔ Quick Tip

The following organizations can provide additional information about seeking care for mental health concerns:

The American Psychiatric
Association
1400 K St., NW
Washington, DC 20005
Phone: 202-682-6000
Fax: 202-682-6850
Website: http://www.psych.org
E-Mail: apa@psych.org

The American Psychological
Association
750 First St., NE
Washington, DC 20002
Toll Free: 800-374-2721
Phone: 202-336-5500
Website: http://www.apa.org

Center for Mental Health
Services
Knowledge Exchange Network
P.O. Box 42490
Washington, DC 20015
Toll-Free: 800-789-2647
Website:
http://www.mentalhealth.org

National Alliance for the
Mentally Ill (NAMI)
2107 Wilson Blvd., Suite 300
Arlington, VA 22201
Toll-Free: 800-950-6264
Fax: 703-524-9094
Website: http://www.nami.org

National Institute of Mental
Health
6001 Executive Boulevard, Rm.
8184, MSC 9663
Rockville, MD 20892-9663
Toll-free 800-64-PANIC
(800-647-2642)
Website:
http://www.nimh.nih.gov

National Mental Health
Association
1021 Prince St.
Alexandria, VA 22314-2971
Toll-Free: 800-969-6642
Website: http://www.nmha.org

How Much Will Therapy Cost?

The cost of treatment depends on many factors including: the type of treatment, the therapist's training, where treatment takes place, and your insurance coverage. The following is a description of typical treatment costs:

Community Mental Health Center: Fees are determined on a sliding scale based on personal income and medical expenses. Fees are set at time of registration and will remain the same whether seen by a social worker, psychiatrist, nurse, or psychologist. Fees range from $5 to $50 per hour. Families covered by medical assistance pay no fee.

Private Clinics: Established fees range from $50 to $100 per hour. Some non-profit agencies have a sliding scale system which may qualify individuals for a lower rate. Fees for group therapy may be lower than for individual therapy.

Private Therapist: Fees generally range from $60 to $125 per hour. Rates for psychologists and psychiatrists are higher than rates for social workers, counselors, and psychiatric nurses.

☞ Remember!!

As you move through the therapeutic process, you should begin to feel gradual relief from your distress, feel more self-assured, and have a greater ability to make decisions and increased comfort in your relationship with others. Therapy may be painful and uncomfortable at times but episodes of discomfort occur during the most successful therapy sessions. Mental health treatment should help you cope with your feelings more effectively.

If you feel you are not getting results, it may be because the treatment you are receiving is not the one best suited to your specific needs. A competent therapist will be eager to discuss your reactions to therapy and respond to your feelings about the process. If you are still dissatisfied, a consultation with another therapist may help you and your therapist evaluate your work.

Hospitalization: Fees for inpatient care range from $400 to $550 per day and vary depending on the setting.

Partial Hospitalization: Typically, day treatment programs are similar to hospital care. Fees range from $95 to $175 per day.

Chapter 44

How Service Agencies Can Help You

There are many helping agencies that provide services for teens. Each one provides a unique service with different philosophies and styles. But there are common things you should know about how you can help an agency best help you.

There are different kinds of help an agency can give you. Some agencies—such as drug and alcohol abuse programs, adoption agencies, or abortion clinics—provide direct help to you and usually cost you some money. Some agencies help you identify the correct agency to go to with your concern. These are called information and referral agencies. They provide their service free to all who call.

Direct services agencies may be paid for and operated in different ways. Some are private, non-profit—this means they have some support from sources other than your payment. They generally can offer sliding scale of fees, meaning that the cost for their service is based upon your ability to pay rather than a pre-set fee for all clients. In a private, for-profit agency, you have to pay a set fee. However, a third party such as your medical insurance sometimes will pay part or all of the costs.

Many agencies have branches near you for service. With others, there is only one office or center that serves your region.

About This Chapter: Text in this chapter is from an undated fact sheet produced and copyrighted by the Children's Hospital for Teens (Akron, Ohio); reprinted with permission.

You should expect to have your concern treated confidentially and with respect. You should expect to receive the same respect and attention as an adult. All birth control agencies will talk confidentially with you without telling your parents (if you are under 18). Other agencies, such as mental health centers, may ask to involve your parents for the help they can give to your treatment.

You should expect that you might be transferred on the phone to several people before your question is completely answered. Do not feel that this is a run-around. The agency just wants to find the best person to help you. Before you call or go to an agency for help, you should prepare by doing a few simple things.

- Get paper and pencil and write down exactly what you want from the agency. Write down your questions, your concerns and any information you need to give to the counselor to help in solving your problem. Do not expect the counselor to automatically know what you want. You must be clear so that they can be clear.

- Keep your paper and pencil with you to write down any information they give to you, such as a contact person's name and phone number. Also, write down and keep a record of the number you called, the person you talked to, the date and time of your call and a summary of your conversation. Do not be afraid to ask the person to slow down or repeat information so that you write it down correctly.

- Be prepared to tell who referred you to the agency you are calling. This will help the counselor know where you have been for help already and how much you already know.

> **☞ Remember!!**
>
> Above all, remember that helping agencies exist to help you. When you contact them you have an opportunity to talk with someone who cares about your concerns.

- Be aware that you will probably talk with a secretary or receptionist first. Their job is field calls, they refer you to the proper counselor. Do not tell your whole story to the secretary. Ask for a specific person, or if you do not know a particular name, ask for intake or the adolescent unit.

Chapter 45

How To Find Help Through Psychotherapy

Millions of Americans have found relief from depression and other emotional difficulties through psychotherapy. Even so, some people find it hard to get started or stay in psychotherapy. This brief question-and-answer guide provides some basic information to help individuals take advantage of outpatient (non-hospital) psychotherapy.

Why Do People Consider Using Psychotherapy?

Psychotherapy is a partnership between an individual and a professional such as a psychologist who is licensed and trained to help people understand their feelings and assist them with changing their behavior. According to the National Institute of Mental Health, one-third of adults in the United States experience an emotional or substance abuse problem. Nearly 25 percent of the adult population suffers at some point from depression or anxiety.

People often consider psychotherapy, also known as therapy, under the following circumstances:

- They feel an overwhelming and prolonged sense of sadness and helplessness, and they lack hope in their lives.

- Their emotional difficulties make it hard for them to function from day to day. For example, they are unable to concentrate on assignments and their job performance suffers as a result.

- Their actions are harmful to themselves or to others. For instance, they drink too much alcohol and become overly aggressive.

- They are troubled by emotional difficulties facing family members or close friends.

✎ Weird Words

Psychoanalysis: A form of psychotherapy in which a patient recalls past experiences as an aid in understanding the unconscious mind. Psychoanalysis is intended to help people learn about the causes of mental and emotional problems.

Psychologist: A professional who is trained to conduct psychological evaluation, therapy, or research. Clinical psychologists must be licensed.

Psychology: The science of studying human behavior and the mind, including its processes and how it is effected by the environment. Psychology is a profession that uses theories about the mind and mental processes to understand and treat a person's problems.

Psychopathology: The study of the nature or causes of mental diseases and behavior disorders.

Psychopharmacology: The study of drugs on the action of the human mind, emotions, and behaviors

Psychotherapy: The treatment of behavioral, emotional, personality, and psychiatric disorders using a variety of psychological methods involving communication between a trained therapist and a person, couple, family, or other group. Forms of psychotherapy include suggestion, hypnotism, and psychoanalysis.

Psychotrophic Drug: A medication that affects the functioning of the mind, behavior, and emotions.

What Does Research Show About The Effectiveness Of Psychotherapy?

Research suggests that therapy effectively decreases patients' depression and anxiety and related symptoms—such as pain, fatigue, and nausea. Psychotherapy has also been found to increase survival time for heart surgery and cancer patients, and it can have a positive effect on the body's immune system. Research increasingly supports the idea that emotional and physical health are very closely linked and that therapy can improve a person's overall health status.

There is convincing evidence that most people who have at least several sessions of psychotherapy are far better off than untreated individuals with emotional difficulties. One major study showed that 50 percent of patients noticeably improved after eight sessions while 75 percent of individuals in psychotherapy improved by the end of six months. Psychotherapy with children is similar in effectiveness to psychotherapy with adults.

How Do I Find A Qualified Therapist?

Selecting a therapist is a highly personal matter.

A professional who works very well with one individual may not be a good choice for another person. There are several ways to get referrals to qualified therapists such as licensed psychologists, including the following:

- Talk to close family members and friends for their recommendations, especially if they have had a good experience with psychotherapy.

- Many state psychological associations operate referral services which put individuals in touch with licensed and competent mental health providers. (Call the American Psychological Association's Practice Directorate at 202-336-5800 for the name and phone number of the appropriate state organization.)

- Ask your primary care physician (or other health professional) for a referral. Tell the doctor what's important to you in choosing a therapist so he or she can make appropriate suggestions.

- Inquire at your church or synagogue.

- Look in the phone book for the listing of a local mental health association or community mental health center and check these sources for possible referrals.

Ideally, you will end up with more than one lead. Call and request the opportunity, either by phone or in person, to ask the therapist some questions. You might want to inquire about his or her licensure and level of training, approach to psychotherapy, participation in insurance plans and fees. Such a discussion should help you sort through your options and choose someone with whom you believe you might interact well.

If I Begin Psychotherapy, How Should I Try To Gain The Most From It?

There are many approaches to outpatient psychotherapy and various formats in which it may occur—including individual, group, and family psychotherapy. Despite the variations, all psychotherapy is a two-way process that works especially well when patients and their therapists communicate openly. Research has shown that the outcome of psychotherapy is improved when the therapist and patient agree early about what the major problems are and how psychotherapy can help.

You and your therapist both have responsibilities in establishing and maintaining a good working relationship. Be clear with your therapist about your expectations and share any concerns that may arise. Psychotherapy works best when you attend all scheduled sessions and give some forethought to what you want to discuss during each one.

How Can I Evaluate Whether Therapy Is Working Well?

As you begin psychotherapy, you should establish clear goals with your therapist. Perhaps you want to overcome feelings of hopelessness associated with depression. Or maybe you would like to control a fear that disrupts your daily life. Keep in mind that certain tasks require more time to accomplish than others. You may need to adjust your goals depending on how long you plan to be in psychotherapy.

After a few sessions, it's a good sign if you feel the experience truly is a joint effort and that you and the therapist enjoy a good rapport. On the other hand, you should be open with your therapist if you find yourself feeling 'stuck' or lacking direction once you've been in psychotherapy awhile.

☞ Remember!!

Psychotherapy isn't easy. But patients who are willing to work in close partnership with their therapist often find relief from their emotional distress and begin to lead more productive and fulfilling lives.

There may be times when a therapist appears cold and disinterested or doesn't seem to regard you positively. Tell your therapist if this is the situation, or if you question other aspects of his or her approach. If you find yourself thinking about discontinuing psychotherapy, talk with your therapist. It might be helpful to consult another professional, provided you let your therapist know you are seeking a second opinion.

Patients often feel a wide range of emotions during psychotherapy. Some qualms about psychotherapy that people may have result from the difficulty of discussing painful and troubling experiences. When this happens, it can actually be a positive sign indicating that you are starting to explore your thoughts and behaviors.

You should spend time with your therapist periodically reviewing your progress (or your concern that you are not making sufficient headway). Although there are other considerations affecting the duration of psychotherapy, success in reaching your primary goals should be a major factor in deciding when your psychotherapy should end.

Chapter 46

How To Start A Self-Help/Advocacy Group

Why Start A Group?

All across the country, self-help/advocacy groups of mental health consumers are springing up. Since the first groups were organized some 15 years ago, this self-help movement has grown to include thousands of consumers, who have organized not only local self-help/advocacy consumer groups but statewide and national organizations as well.

This vast network started with a few people who had the idea of getting together with others who, like themselves, had experienced psychiatric hospitalization. They were seeking emotional support, information about mental health issues, individual advocacy, and a way to improve the mental health system. They were also looking for others to join with them in the fight against the stigma of mental illness and against the economic and social discrimination faced by those with psychiatric histories. They also hoped to find friends. They found everything they were looking for.

Where Do You Begin?

You begin at the beginning, with the desire to start a self-help/advocacy group of mental health consumers. Like all good things, a group can begin

About This Chapter: Text in this chapter is from an undated document titled "How to Start a Self-Help/Advocacy Group," by Joseph A. Rogers, produced by the National Mental Health Consumers' Self-Help Clearinghouse with funding from the Community Support Program of the Center for Mental Health Services (CMHS); reprinted with permission.

with one person with an idea. You don't even need to know what you'd like the group to accomplish; at this stage, you can concentrate on bringing people together—goals can wait. People have started self-help groups simply out of a wish to find other people who have had similar experiences.

Once you've got the idea, it's important to find at least one or two other people who have the same idea, or whom you can sell on the idea of starting a group. It's very difficult to start something entirely by yourself; it's a good idea to have someone with whom to share the work and discuss your plans. Finding these other people may be as simple as asking a couple of your friends who have been through the same experiences you have if they want to start a self-help group.

> ✎ **Weird Words**
>
> Advocacy: Efforts made on behalf of the patient representing his or her the needs.

If you don't know any people you can interest in the idea, you might try putting an ad in the newspaper. In fact, many newspapers have a free "bulletin board" column where you can list events; your meeting would qualify. Or you might ask local service providers if they'll put a notice up. The providers might include the Community Mental Health Center (CMHC), a minister, doctor or social worker. Notices can also be posted, with permission, in unemployment offices, Laundromats, 7-11's—any place that people might see them. These notices only have to say that so-and-so at such-and-such a phone number is interested in starting a self-help group for present and former mental patients (or mental health consumers, etc.) and invite anyone who may be interested in such a group to call. Another way to find interested people is to network: Talk to everyone you know and get the news out by word of mouth; the grapevine often bears fruit.

One relatively easy way to identify interested people is to attend meetings of any mental health advocates, mental health workers, or family groups, or attend conferences, speeches or other presentations where other consumers are present. You might ask the speaker if you can announce the formation of a self-help group before or after their presentation; they'll be delighted to agree. Then, with everyone's attention, you can ask interested people to come up and give you their names and phone numbers after the meeting. Then you can contact them when you have set up a time and place for your first meeting.

Your First Meeting

Your first meeting can usually be arranged very easily, especially if it only involves the few individuals who are planning the group's development. Most groups start very slowly and grow over time, so don't get disappointed if you only have two or three members at first. Even if your group starts with just you and a couple of friends, that is enough to begin with: A small group can still accomplish important work.

You might ask for space at the local community mental health center to hold your first planning meeting. If there are clients at the center who want to become involved, this gives them the opportunity to meet at a familiar place. And you'll have the benefit of inertia in attracting participants.

If you are meeting in a Community Mental Health Center, it is important to make it clear that the group is independent and that fees should not be charged and no names should be taken by staff. This is not a mental health center program. Staff should not run or dominate the meeting: this is self-help! Staff can help start or facilitate the meeting or group, provided everyone is clear that their role then is to withdraw and let consumers take over.

You may find—especially if you live in a rural area—that the local CMHC is the only space available. So use these facilities if you must, but view it as temporary and find other space as soon as you can.

At the beginning, it's sometimes easier to meet at a local diner, where you can begin the early stages of planning a group over a cup of coffee and not have to worry about finding a meeting place. In fact, one group in Miami, Florida, started out meeting in diners, and they're still doing it. Sometimes, for the price of a cup of coffee or a bowl of soup, a restaurant will let you meet in a private back room, if they have the space available and they're not too busy.

You may need to have the group meet in the daytime to allow for travel time. Unless you're in a city, you may need to cover a large area to attract more than a few consumers. But other consumer groups in large, rural states have had the same problems of overcoming time, distance and cost, and have managed to get their groups going. You may need to spend more initial time talking one-on-one with consumers to ensure their involvement, or more time talking/advertising to local mental health centers to make contacts.

Do Professionals Have A Place In Self-Help?

As mentioned above, professional involvement in self-help can be tricky. Even the most progressive mental health professionals may hold attitudes and prejudices, albeit unconsciously, that may stand in the way when their clients try to develop a truly independent self-help group. It can also be difficult for clients to deal with a professional in a consulting role. In the past, most programs encouraged clients to be the recipients of services, instead of a co-producer of their own support systems. Too often, this is still the case.

Because of this, many ex-patients believe that the only role of the professional mental health system in self-help should be as a funding source. As one mental health consumer put it, "If professionals are involved, then it's not self-help." But the professional who truly believes in consumer empowerment can be of considerable assistance in getting a group started. For example, many consumers have never heard of the self-help movement. The professional can be a transmitter of knowledge, to get the word out that the self-help movement exists.

The professional's role should evolve from one of greater to lesser participation—ideally, to total disengagement. At the beginning, the professional can be a conduit of information. He or she can talk to clients about the self-help movement, tell them about movement publications, and invite consultants from other groups to speak. If the clients show an interest, the professional may take the next step and become an initiator, perhaps calling the first meeting.

Once a group has begun to meet, the professional's role should change from initiator to facilitator. It's important that the consumers take the leadership;

the professional should encourage this. After the group has gained some momentum, the professional must take another step backward and become a consultant, "on call" in case the group wants outside assistance. He or she may keep in touch, even attend occasional meetings if invited, but must wait for an invitation before intervening in any way.

The First LARGE Meeting

Once you have been able to find one or two other individuals who are interested in starting a self-help group and are willing to put in some effort to get it off the ground so that the entire burden does not rest on any one individual, the next step is to plan your first large public meeting. This does not mean a cast of thousands—we're talking about trying to attract at least six or seven or ten or twenty people.

It's a good idea to find a neutral and comfortable meeting place in the community. You may find that your local library, church, or school already offers meeting places to other self-help groups, and wouldn't mind adding yours to the list. Ask your local chapter of Alcoholics Anonymous where their groups meet; the same churches or other public meeting places will probably be willing to offer your group the same hospitality.

Some places may charge a fee. If you can't afford this, you can usually—especially with churches—work out an arrangement where your group would do some "in-kind" service—painting a wall, raking the yard, etc.—to compensate for your use of the building. Other good possibilities are organizations like the Kiwanis and Lions and Veterans of Foreign Wars. These groups will sometimes offer meeting places at very low cost, if not absolutely free. Also, try municipal buildings, such as City Hall chambers, firehouses and town recreation centers—any places that the town officials may make available to their citizens.

You can always meet in each other's homes. This is fairly easy in the early stage, but if you want to publicize your group, it becomes more complicated. Some members may not wish to have their names and addresses included in an announcement of a self help meeting for mental health consumers.

What you are looking for is a relatively small, comfortable, private room, where people aren't going to be constantly walking through. It would be great to find a room without an institutional atmosphere, although that may be difficult if you're choosing among classrooms, firehouses and municipal meeting rooms. However, a lot of churches have small, cozy rooms that they make available to groups.

Setting The Tone

Your small organizing committee of one or two other people should plan your initial group meeting. This is the meeting that will set the tone for at least the next few meetings. What you're trying to do is spark the group's growth so that you're able to accomplish some of the goals you had in mind when you had the idea of starting a self-help group in the first place.

At this initial meeting, start to open the planning process up to the new participants. It's all too easy to get into a situation where the two or three people who have been involved from the beginning have some strong ideas about the group's goals, and consider the first meeting a forum for announcing their goals to the large group. This is a serious pitfall. Since the hope is to involve as many people in the work as possible—since this is what gives the group its "strength in numbers"—going in with your agenda carved in stone can only discourage the new arrivals.

Therefore, although it's fine for the planning committee to have some clear ideas about its goals, it's important to solicit from the people who are newly involved what their own goals are and how they think the group should function. This will give these people a sense of ownership, of belonging to the group.

Brainstorming

You might bring in a blackboard or an easel with a large newsprint pad. After some orientation by the planning committee, ask each of the attendees to give at least one goal, one activity, one "Thing" they would like to get out of the group, and list these on the board. Usually, during this Brainstorming session you should not criticize or eliminate anybody's suggestions.

Among the goals people focus on have been their concerns about the conditions at the local state hospitals or CMHCs; problems with their medications or treatment; interest in learning about advocacy and their legal rights; concerns about the lack of community treatment services, housing, employment or benefits, or about discrimination in these areas; or their need for social and recreational opportunities.

After everyone has had a chance to have his or her goals listed, the group can narrow them down to the ones that a majority of the people involved agree upon. Later, the group can develop an "action plan" to work on achieving these goals.

You'll find that most people have pretty much the same ideas as you do about the purpose of a self-help group. But be open to other ideas; don't be critical just because they're different from yours. The group should be a "group effort." If some goals seem very unrealistic, or if the only group members in favor of them are the people who suggested them, some time might be merited in discussing how you can reach an agreement on the one or two goals everyone may have in common.

Sharing

During this first meeting, it's important to establish that the group is open to everyone's participation, and that the work must be shared. Although two or three individuals have done the lion's share of the work of getting the group going until now, a lot of these tasks now need to be divided among the whole group.

Don't be disappointed if at first it seems that the same two or three people are doing all the work. It takes a while for people to decide that anything is worth investing much time or energy in. It may be two or three meetings or more before you're able to get people to handle some of the tasks that your planning committee has been taking care of.

Even from the beginning, it's good to list tasks as they relate to the goals the group has discussed. Demonstrate that there is a connection between tasks and achieving goats, and that everyone should pitch in, even if it's about something as simple as refreshments for the next meeting. There's always a lot of work to be done in a group; the more that work is shared, the more people feel a sense of participation. But again, don't be disappointed if it takes a while for this to happen.

It also may take a while to get people to focus on specific issues. In fact, they may not even get to this in the initial meeting. But it's your job as facilitator to try to keep the meeting running smoothly. From the beginning, establish some ground rules on how to keep the discussion moving. Some groups find it easier to use already established ground rules of other self-help groups; ask other local organizations about how they handle meetings. But you do have an important role in keeping the flow going and making sure everybody has a chance to speak—that no one dominates the meeting.

Agenda

Before the first meeting, plan to divide the time equally between business—when you are explaining the group and establishing ground rules as well as discussing possible goals and assigning tasks—and pleasure, a time for socializing. Ninety minutes is about the most that people want to participate in a formal group structure. So allocate 45 minutes or so to business and use the rest of the time for socializing. It's a good idea to have refreshments—at least some cookies and coffee or fruit juice—since eating always makes people feel more comfortable.

Finally, remember that all of us have had both successes and problems starting our groups. In spite of your hard work, sometimes the number of people who show up and get involved will be very small. But your work is never really wasted: Every person you have contacted is a potential member someday. Also, you may have helped to erase some of the stigma of mental illness just by trying to start a group.

If you have tried to start a group but could not get one going, you may want to put the idea on hold for a few months. Another new game plan—after all, football teams often change strategies at half time—is to try to find a worthwhile project or two that you can do with the people you have. Some other options are to reach out to other consumer groups in other areas, states or nationally for advice, support, and ideas. More and more consumer groups are having their own conferences and meetings to network with new groups and members.

The Next Meeting

Don't forget to get everybody's name and phone number, and give out the name and number of a contact person. Also establish when your regular meeting time and place will be so that everyone can plan for it. Most groups find that a weekly meeting is about the most they can handle; some groups meet every other week. If you do meet every other week, make it a regular intervals, such as the first and third Wednesday of the month, or the second and fourth Thursday. This way, it's a regular time and people can plan for it.

As your group begins to grow, you may want to think about linking up in a statewide network. Your state may already have a network of consumer groups. (You can find this out by contacting the Clearinghouse.)

Another way to link up with other consumers is to attend national conferences, such as the annual Alternatives conferences or the National Mental Health Consumer Leadership Training Institute, or regional Community Support Program conferences near your home state. There are other statewide and local consumer and coalition conferences that are being held more and more frequently. (You can also get in touch with the Clearinghouse to find about conferences.)

Other Sources Of Information

1. Hill, Karen, *Helping You Helps Me*, Canadian Council on Social Development, 1987.

2. Stroul, Beth A., *Models of Community Support Services*, National Institute of Mental Health, 1986.

3. Humm, Andy, *How to Organize a Self-Help Group*, National Self-Help Clearinghouse, New York 1979.

4. Katz, Fred, and Eugene Bender, *The Strength in Us*, New Viewpoints, New York 1976.

5. Gartner, Alan, and Frank Riessman, *Help: A Working Guide to Self-Help Groups*, New Viewpoints, New York.

6. Silverman, Phyllis, *Mutual Help Groups: Organization and Development*, Sage Publications, 1980.

7. Mallow, Lucretia, *Leading Self-Help Groups: A Guide for Training Facilitators*, Family Service America, 1984.

The National Mental Health Consumers' Self-Help Clearinghouse

1211 Chestnut Street, Suite 1207
Philadelphia, PA 19107
Toll-Free: 800-533-4539
Phone: 215-751-1810
Fax: 215-636-6312
Website: http://www.mhselfhelp.org
E-Mail: info@mhselfhelp.org

Chapter 47

Medications Used In Treatment

Medications For Mood Disorders

Effective medical treatments now exist for the full range of mood disorders, from mild depression to severe manic depression. Treatment decisions are based on the severity of the symptoms as well as the type of symptomatology. There are a wide variety of treatments that are now available, but research studies consistently demonstrate that combined psychotherapy and medication treatments produce the best results. The psychotherapy treatments work by helping with the psychosocial and interpersonal adjustment of the individual, whereas the drugs help with the physical and physiologically based symptoms. Psychotherapy seems to help by improving the patient's willingness to continue with the medication treatment, also.

This section will focus on psychopharmacological treatments for depression and manic depression. Although the mode of action of the various psychotropic medications is not precisely known, it is thought that these drugs work by correcting imbalances in the brain's chemical messenger or neurotransmitter system. The brain is a highly complex organ, and it may be

About This Chapter: Information about medications for mood disorders is from "Pharmacological Treatment of Mood Disorders," by David M. Goldstein, M.D., Director, Mood Disorders Program, Georgetown University Medical Center, © Depression and Related Affective Disorders Association (DRADA); reprinted with permission. Information about medications for anxiety disorders is from "What Medications Are Used to Treat Anxiety Disorders," © 1999 Anxiety Disorders Association of America. Reprinted with permission of the Anxiety Disorders Association of America.

✎ Weird Words

<u>Dopamine:</u> A chemical found in the body that acts as a neurotransmitter and is involved with some movement disorders and some forms of mental illness in which the patient experiences a loss of contact with reality.

<u>Efficacy:</u> The ability of a drug or other type of therapy to bring about a wanted result; to be effective.

<u>Neurotransmitter:</u> A specific body chemical that aids or inhibits the transmission of impulses between two nerve cells; examples are dopamine and norepinephrine.

<u>Norepinephrine:</u> A hormone that causes constriction of blood vessels and raises blood pressure; it is secreted in response to low blood pressure and stress. Mood disorders are believed to be linked to disturbances of the metabolism of norepinephrine in the brain.

<u>Psychopharmacology:</u> The study of drugs on the action of the human mind, emotions, and behaviors.

<u>Psychotic:</u> Associated with psychosis, which is the loss of contact with reality, delusions, or hallucinations.

<u>Psychotrophic Drug:</u> A medication that affects the functioning of the mind, behavior, and emotions.

<u>Serotonin:</u> A body chemical that stimulates smooth muscle contraction, inhibits gastric (stomach) secretions, and works as a central neurotransmitter. Serotonin is important in sleep cycles.

<u>Side Effect:</u> An effect other than the therapeutic effect for which a drug or therapy is given. Side effects are usually—but not always—undesirable. Common side effects include nausea and headaches.

<u>Symptomatology:</u> The combined total of all of the symptoms related to a disease.

that the medications work to restore normal regulatory processes in the brain. These drugs are quite effective if taken for sufficient lengths of time and at proper dosages. It is common for there to be a several week delay in the onset of effectiveness of the medication, so patience and cooperation with the prescribing physician are crucial elements in treatment. A primary cause of patients' noncompliance with medication treatment is the emergence of side effects. The side effects associated with the use of these medications generally are dependent upon dosage and duration of treatment. A close, cooperative, and trusting relationship with the physician is important in helping the individual to navigate through the side effects, should they occur.

These medications have been carefully studied and have to pass rigorous standards by the U.S. Food and Drug Administration (FDA) in order to be released into the marketplace. All available antidepressant prescription medications have been found to be safe and effective and they are not known to be addictive.

Medication choice is guided by diagnosis, so before treatment begins, care must be taken to accurately diagnose the medical condition that best explains the presenting symptoms. Treatments for depression and manic depression often differ and this is an important distinction. Manic depressive patients treated with antidepressants alone may be at an increased risk for the development of a manic episode.

Medication For Depression

There are over thirty antidepressant medications now available in the United States to treat depression. There are three principal neurotransmitters that are involved in the development of depression, and they are serotonin, norepinephrine, and dopamine. The available antidepressant medications differ in which of these neurotransmitters are affected. The medications also differ in which side-effects they are likely to induce. Other differences among the medications involve how they interact with other medications that an individual might be taking. The medications for depression can be categorized in the following way:

- Heterocyclic antidepressants
- Monoamine oxidase inhibitors (MOAIs)
- Selective serotonin reuptake inhibitors (SSRIs)

Heterocylic antidepressants: The heterocyclic antidepressants were the mainstay of antidepressant treatment from their inception in the United States in the late 1950s until the mid 1980s. These drugs include the tricyclic antidepressants, such as Elavil, Tofranil, Pamelor, Norpramin, and Vivactil. These medications have been quite effective in improving the symptoms of depression, but their usefulness is limited by the associated side-effects. These side-effects include dry mouth, constipation, weight gain, urinary hesitancy, rapid heartbeat, and dizziness upon arising. These side-effects, although they are rarely dangerous, may be of significant magnitude to warrant stopping that medication and switching to another. A more recent member of the heterocyclic family is a new medication named Remeron. This is a recently released antidepressant that is chemically similar to the older compounds, although it has a more favorable side-effect profile.

Monoamine oxidase inhibitor antidepressants (MAO inhibitors): The monoamine oxidase inhibitor antidepressants, or MAOIs, are a group of antidepressants that were developed in the 1950s also. Initially they were used as treatments for tuberculosis, but were discovered to have antidepressant properties among that population. These medications can be highly effective for some individuals who have what is referred to as "atypical depression." These are patients who have a dominance of fatigue, excessive need for sleep, weight gain, and rejection sensitivity. Some investigators feel that this group of patients respond preferentially to MAOI drugs. This category of medications includes drugs such as Nardil and Parnate. Monoamine oxidase inhibitor drugs are limited by the possibility of the infrequent but at times life threatening side effect of hypertensive crisis. This is a phenomenon where, while taking the medication, the individual eats certain foodstuffs or takes certain medications that contain an amino acid known as tyramine. This results in a sudden and severe rise in blood pressure associated with a severe headache. In some instances the use of this medication can be extremely helpful, but the dietary restrictions have to be followed faithfully.

Selective serotonin reuptake inhibitors (SSRIs): The final category of antidepressant medication is known as the selective serotonin reuptake inhibitors, or SSRI drugs. The first of these agents was Prozac, which came on the market in 1987, and was followed in short order by Zoloft, Paxil, Luvox, and more recently by Effexor and Serzone. Another medication related to this group is Wellbutrin. This group of medications has been shown to be equally effective in treating depression as compared to the older heterocyclic and MAOI medications. The advantage of these drugs is that they have fewer and more benign side effects. Generally speaking, they have fewer cardiovascular side effects and present fewer problems to the patients or the physician. They are not without side effects, however, and some patients report symptoms such as nausea, sexual inhibition, insomnia, weight gain, and daytime sedation.

Results Of Treatment

Approximately 60-70% of patients who present with symptoms of depression will be successfully treated by the first antidepressant that they take. The remaining 30% of individuals may be helped by trying a second, third, or even fourth medication. In certain instances, the physician may enhance the effectiveness of a particular drug by adding on other agents, such as lithium, thyroid supplementation, or a second antidepressant concurrent with the initial medication. There are difficulties that may develop with loss of efficacy of antidepressants, also. In approximately 20% of cases, individual antidepressants seem to lose their efficacy. When this happens, the physician may change medication or try one of the enhancement strategies suggested above.

Medication For Manic Depressive Illness (Bipolar Disorder)

Lithium: The first treatment developed for manic depressive illness was lithium carbonate. Lithium is a naturally occurring mineral that was known in the 19th century to have positive effects on mood. In the late 1940s it was evaluated by a psychiatrist in Australia and found to have beneficial effects in manic depressive illness. This research was followed up in the 1950s by Dr. Morgens Schou in Scandinavia. Since that time, lithium has been the mainstay of treatment for manic depressive illness, being effective for both the manic as well as the depressed phases of that illness. Lithium may be taken alone or in conjunction with other medications, depending on the circumstances. Side effects of lithium treatment include weight gain, memory impairment, tremor, acne, and occasionally thyroid dysfunction. During treatment with lithium, which is usually over an extended period of time, that patient should be monitored for thyroid function as well as kidney function.

Valproic acid (Depakote): In addition to lithium, there are a number of other agents available for treatment of manic depressive illness. Valproic acid is commonly prescribed as Depakote, and is an effective agent for mood stabilization. Current research studies are underway to compare the efficacy of Depakote as compared to lithium. Side effects associated with Depakote include nausea, weight gain, hair loss, and increased bruising.

Carbamazepine (Tegretol): A third commonly used mood stabilizer is Tegretol. This is a medication that was initially developed for facial pain and subsequently found to be useful for certain types of epilepsy. In the past twenty years it has been developed as a mood stabilizer, and it has been found to have anti-manic, antidepressant, and prophylactic efficacy. Tegretol is associated with a relatively low incidence of weight gain, memory loss, and nausea. Skin rash is sometimes found with Tegretol, and there is the

---

✔ Quick Tip

Continuing Or Discontinuing Medications For Mood Disorders

Depression and manic depression tend to be recurrent problems, and often maintenance medication is recommended. This recommendation should be discussed carefully between the patient and his or her physician.

Another issue in the use of the psychotropic medications is the issue of discontinuation. The timing of discontinuation of psychotropic medications is an important and highly individual decision, which should always be made in conjunction with one's physician. As a general rule, stopping medications in a gradual way is preferable to abrupt discontinuation. Abrupt discontinuation may result in return of original

possibility of bone marrow suppression, which requires monitoring by blood tests.

New medications: There have been several new medications that are under development for the treatment of manic depressive illness and show some promise. Neurontin, or gabapentin is an anticonvulsant compound which is being developed as a mood stabilizer. It shows promise and has the benefit of very few interactions with other medications. Another medication under development is Lamictal. This medication is an anticonvulsant, approved in the United States as an anticonvulsant several years ago. It has been found to have antidepressant properties, and may turn out to have mood stabilizing effects as well, although this is currently under investigation. Lamictal carries the risk of rash with it, which at times may be severe.

Antipsychotic Medications

Antipsychotic medications have usefulness in more severe states of depression and manic depression. This group of medications is very effective in

symptoms, or may result in what is referred to as "discontinuation syndrome." Discontinuation syndrome has a variable presentation. Patients often will feel as if they have a severe case of the flu. Abrupt discontinuation of lithium in the context of manic depressive illness carries the risk of a sudden return of manic or depressive symptomatology. In addition, there is a small group of manic depressive patients who, once they discontinue lithium, become resistant to its effectiveness at a later time.

These medications can be highly effective and may significantly alter the course of an individual's life. One must always keep in mind that the choice to take the medication is based on an assessment of the risks and benefits associated with taking medication as well as not taking the medication. Those choices should always be undertaken in the context of an ongoing relationship with the prescribing physician.

controlling severe agitation, disorganization, as well as psychotic symptoms which sometimes accompany the more severe instances of mood
disorders.

Typical antipsychotic medications: The typical antipsychotic medications
include drugs such as Haldol, Trilafon, Stelazine, and Mellaril. They are quite
effective in controlling agitation as well as hallucinations and unrealistic
thoughts. They are less effective in controlling or treating the apathy, withdrawal, and indifference that sometimes occurs in these conditions. (Individuals with mood disorders may have an increased potential for developing
neurological side effects associated with the use of these medications, specifically a condition referred to as Tardive Dyskinesia. This is a persistent
twitching of the fingers or lips.)

Atypical antipsychotic medications: In recent years, a new class of
antipsychotics has become available referred to as the "Atypical antipsychotic
medications." This includes Clozaril, Zyprexa, and Risperdal. This group of
medications represents an advance over the older medications in that they
continue to be effective against psychotic symptoms such as agitation and
hallucinations, but they are also helpful in treating apathy and indifference
which may also occur. These medications seem to have a significantly reduced likelihood of development of neurological side effects as well.

What Medications Are Used To Treat Anxiety Disorders?

Azaspirones: Azaspirones is a class of drug effective in the treatment of
generalized anxiety disorder (GAD). It works gradually over 2-4 weeks to
relieve symptoms of GAD. It does not cause sedation, impair memory or
balance, nor does it increase the effects of alcohol. It is not habit forming and
can be discontinued without causing withdrawal symptoms. The drug is generally well tolerated and the side effects are not usually serious enough to
make most people stop taking it.

Benzodiazepines: Most of the benzodiazepines are effective against generalized anxiety disorder (GAD). Some drugs in this group are also used to
treat panic disorder and social phobia.

Benzodiazepines are relatively fast-acting drugs. Their principal side effect is drowsiness, but they have the potential for dependency. Individuals taking benzodiazepines can experience a return of their anxiety symptoms when the drug is discontinued. They may also experience temporary withdrawal symptoms. These problems can be minimized if the patient and doctor work together.

Beta blockers: These drugs are used mainly to reduce certain anxiety symptoms like palpitations, sweating and tremors, and to control anxiety in public situations. They often are prescribed for individuals with social phobia. Beta blockers reduce blood pressure and slow the heartbeat.

Tricyclics (TCAs): These drugs were first used for treating depression, but some are also effective in blocking panic attacks. Most tricyclics may also reduce symptoms of post-traumatic stress disorder (PTSD) and some are effective against obsessive-compulsive disorder (OCD).

Tricyclics generally take two or three weeks to take effect. Some individuals feel the drugs' most annoying side effect is weight gain. Other side effects include drowsiness, dry mouth, dizziness and impaired sexual function.

Monoamine Oxidase Inhibitors (MAOIs): These drugs are used in the treatment of panic disorder, social phobia, PTSD and sometimes OCD, but they require dietary restrictions and some doctors prefer to try other treatments first. Anyone taking a MAO inhibitor must avoid other medications, wine and beer, and food such as cheeses that contain tyramine.

Serotonin Reuptake Inhibitors (SRIs): These are the newest medicines available for treating anxiety disorders. SRIs may be considered a first-line of treatment for panic disorder, and they often are effective against obsessive-compulsive disorder (OCD). Traditionally used to treat depression, the safety and convenience of SRIs (they require once-a-day dosing) have made them among the most widely-used drugs in the world. The most common side effect, which tends to resolve over time, is mild nausea. Sexual dysfunction also has been reported.

New medications: New medications are being developed and tested constantly. Your doctor will advise you if one of these newer drugs is appropriate.

✔ Quick Tip

For more information about medications for depression, bipolar disorder, or other mood disorders, contact:

Depression and Related Disorders Association
Meyer 3-181, 550 Bldg.
600 North Wolfe Street
Baltimore, MD 21287-7381
Phone: 410-955-4647
Fax: 410-614-3241
Website: http://www.med.jhu.edu/drada

For more information about medications for anxiety disorders, contact:

Anxiety Disorders Association of America (ADAA)
11900 Parklawn Drive, Suite 100
Rockville, MD 20852
Phone: 301-231-9350
Fax: 301-231-7392
Website: http://www.adaa.org
E-Mail: AnxDis@adaa.org

Chapter 48

What About St. John's Wort?

Introduction

St. John's wort (*Hypericum perforatum*) is a long-living, wild-growing herb with yellow flowers that has been used for centuries to treat mental disorders as well as nerve pain. In ancient times, doctors and herbalists (herb specialists) wrote about its use as a sedative and antimalarial agent as well as a balm for wounds, burns, and insect bites. Today, the herb is a popular treatment for mild to moderate depression; it also is used to treat anxiety, seasonal affective disorder, and sleep disorders.[1]

St. John's wort is most widely used in Germany, where doctors prescribed almost 66 million daily doses in 1994 for psychological complaints.[2] In fact, German doctors prescribe St. John's wort about 20 times more often than Prozac, one of the most widely prescribed antidepressants in the United States.[3]

The use of St. John's wort is growing in the United States, and several brands now are available. Extracts of the plant are sold as a nutritional

About This Chapter: Text in this chapter is from "St. John's Wort Fact Sheet," produced by the National Center for Complementary and Alternative Medicine (NCCAM), a component of the National Institutes of Health (NIH), Publication Z-02, April 1999. This version is from the NCCAM Web site (http://nccam.nih.gov/nccam); it was updated in October 1999. Inclusion of a treatment or resource does not imply endorsement by the National Center for Complementary and Alternative Medicine, National Institutes of Health, or U.S. Public Health Service.

supplement after being prepared with a powder or an oil; the herb is available in capsule, tea, or tincture forms. St. John's wort was among the top-selling botanical products in the United States in 1997, with industry-estimated sales of $400 million in 1998.[4]

U.S. Food And Drug Administration's Role

St. John's wort is 1 of 200 plant products approved by the U.S. Food and Drug Administration (FDA) for sale to the public as a dietary supplement. The FDA does not subject dietary supplements to an extensive premarket approval process, however, as it does new drugs.[5] On the other hand, the Dietary Supplement Health and Education Act of 1994 permits the FDA to remove a supplement from the market if it determines the supplement is unsafe. Herbal products such as St. John's wort can be marketed without stating standards for dosage or evidence of safety. Often, information on specific products may be misleading or even inaccurate. For instance, when the *Los Angeles Times*, a newspaper in California, commissioned laboratory tests on 10 St. John's wort products, researchers found that the potency of the products varied dramatically from what their labels claimed.[6]

At the same time, a St. John's wort product stating the words "standardized extract" in its label may be more likely to contain the exact amount of the specific active ingredient needed to be effective. Standardized products generally are considered the highest-quality herbal products that a consumer can buy.[7]

Treating Depression

Depression is a common illness that strikes perhaps 1 in 15 Americans each year. A person's mood, thoughts, physical health, and behavior all may be affected.

> ✎ **Weird Words**
>
> Antidepressant: Medication or other therapy used to counteract depression.
>
> Herb: A soft-stemmed plant used in as seasoning and in medicine.
>
> Side Effect: An effect other than the therapeutic effect for which a drug or therapy is given. Side effects are usually—but not always—undesirable. Common side effects include nausea and headaches.

Symptoms can include a persistent sad, anxious, or "empty" feeling; loss of energy, appetite, or sexual drive; and lack of interest in socializing, work, or hobbies.

Depression can be mild, moderate, or severe. Mild depression is characterized by difficulty in functioning normally, while moderate depression may involve impaired functioning at work or in social activities. Severe depression, which may involve delusions or hallucinations, markedly interferes with a person's ability to work or otherwise function and may lead to suicide. Genetic factors may put a person at risk for developing depression, and alcohol or drug use can make the problem worse.[8] While the public misperception persists that depression is voluntary or a "character flaw," depression is a real condition that can be treated effectively by qualified professionals.[9]

Specific psychotherapies (such as interpersonal and cognitive-behavioral therapy) and antidepressant medications both have been found to be effective for patients with major depression. Major depression includes mild, moderate, or severe depression that is not characterized by manic-depressive mood swings or induced by a substance such as alcohol. Several antidepressant drugs have become more widely used in the past several years and been found to be effective. However, patients sometimes report unpleasant side effects such as a dry mouth, nausea, headache, diarrhea, or impaired sexual function or sleep.[10]

In part because of these types of drug side effects, many patients with depression are turning to herbal treatments such as St. John's wort. Researchers are studying it for possibly having fewer and less severe side effects than antidepressant drugs. St. John's wort also costs far less than antidepressant medication. In addition, St. John's wort does not require a prescription.[11]

St. John's wort is not completely free of side effects, however. Some users have complained of a dry mouth, dizziness, gastrointestinal symptoms, increased sensitivity to sunlight, and fatigue.[12] In addition, herbal treatments often are not as potent or as quick to act as conventional treatments. Furthermore, herbal treatments may not produce the desired results and may not be as effective as conventional medicine. Still, some people turn to herbs because they prefer to use "natural" products.

✤ It's A Fact!!

How St. John's Wort Works

The major components in extracts of St. John's wort include flavonoids, kaempferol, luteolin, biapigenin, hyperforin, polycyclic phenols, hypericin, and pseudohypericin. Researchers believe the last three substances are the active ingredients.[5] New research suggests that hyperforin also may play a large role in the herb's antidepressant effects. Some German manufacturers of St. John's wort have begun standardizing, not only to hypericin as most U.S. manufacturers do, but to hyperforin as well.[13] Standardizing means that the manufacturer ensures that each individual supplement contains a uniform amount of a certain compound, in this case hypericin and hyperforin.

Recent research suggests a possible application of St. John's wort for alcoholism. Researchers from the University of North Carolina at Chapel Hill found that St. John's wort reduced alcohol intake in laboratory animals.[14]

Several mechanisms of action of St. John's wort have been proposed, including the following:

- Inhibition of monoamine (serotonin, dopamine, and norepinephrine) re-uptake: St. John's wort appears to reduce the rate at which brain cells reabsorb serotonin (an important neurotransmitter or chemical that aids communication between nerve cells). Low levels of serotonin in the body are associated with depression.[15,16]

- Modulation of interleukin-6 (IL-6) activity: Raised levels of IL-6, a protein involved in the communication between cells in the body's immune (disease-fighting) system, may lead to increases in adrenal regulatory hormones, a hallmark of depression. St. John's wort may reduce levels of IL-6, and thus help treat depression.[17]

More research is needed to determine precisely the active ingredients in St. John's wort and to learn how the herb works.

Clinical depression is a serious medical disorder that, in many cases, can be treated. However, St. John's wort is not a proven therapy for clinical depression. Therefore, there is some risk in taking it to treat clinical depression.[5]

In any case, St. John's wort should not be mixed with other standard antidepressants because side effects may result. This is one reason why it is important to tell your doctor about all medications you are taking. Check with your doctor before taking St. John's wort or any other herb or medication. Your doctor can help you weigh the risks and benefits of a particular treatment so you can make informed health care decisions.

Clinical Trials

Clinical trials (studies of a treatment's safety and effectiveness in humans) have found a similar rate of response with St. John's wort as with standard, conventional antidepressants in treating mild to moderate depression.[18,19] However, it is hard to interpret these studies as definite proof of the efficacy of St. John's wort because low doses of standard antidepressants were used and there was no placebo (a pharmacologically inactive substance) control. An analysis of 23 European clinical studies of St. John's wort that was published in the *British Medical Journal* in 1996 concluded that the herb has antidepressive effects in cases of mild to moderate depression (the dosage varied considerably among the studies).[2] However, no studies of its long-term use have been conducted. More research is needed to explore the long-term effects and optimum safe dosage of the extract.

A new study funded by the National Institutes of Health's National Center for Complementary and Alternative Medicine (NCCAM), Office of Dietary Supplements, and the National Institute of Mental Health will provide more information about St. John's wort. This study, which is in progress, is the first large-scale controlled clinical trial in the United States to assess whether the herb has a significant therapeutic effect in patients with clinical depression. The $4.3 million study will involve 336 patients with major depression. The Duke University Medical Center in Durham, North Carolina, is coordinating the 3-year study, which has 13 clinical sites around the country.

There are three different treatment groups in the trial. One group will receive an initial dose of 900 mg per day of St. John's wort; a second will receive a placebo; and the third will receive Zoloft (a commonly used antidepressant). Patients who respond positively to their randomly assigned treatment will be continued on it for another 4 months.

References

1. American Herbal Pharmacopoeia and Therapeutic Compendium. "St. John's Wort (*Hypericum perforatum*) Monograph." Herbalgram. *The Journal of the American Botanical Council and the Herb Research Foundation.* 1997. (40):1-16.

2. Linde, K., Ramirez, G., Mulrow, C.D., Weidenhammer, W., and Melchart, D. "St. John's Wort for Depression—An Overview and Metaanalysis of Randomized Clinical Trials." *British Medical Journal.* 1996. 313(7052):253-8.

3. Murray, M. "Common Questions About St. John's Wort Extract." *American Journal of Natural Medicine.* 1997. 4(7):14-9.

4. *Nutrition Business Journal.* San Diego, CA: Nutrition Business International, 1998.

☞ **Remember!!**

If you need more information about depression, contact the National Institute of Mental Health toll-free at 1-800-421-4211. For more information about St. John's wort, contact the American Botanical Council at 512-926-4900 or the Herb Research Foundation at 303-449-2265. For more information about complementary and alternative medicine, contact the NCCAM Clearinghouse at 1-888-644-6226.

Please send requests for information about complementary or alternative medicine to:

NCCAM Clearinghouse
P.O. Box 8218
Silver Spring, MD 20907-8218
Phone: 1-888-644-6226 (1-888-NIH-NCAM) (Toll-Free, TTY/TDY, Fax-On-Demand)
Fax: 1-301-495-4957
E-mail: nccamc@altmedinfo.org
Web site: http://nccam.nih.gov/nccam

5. National Institute of Mental Health. "Questions and Answers About St. John's Wort," Bethesda, MD: National Institute of Mental Health, 1997.

6. Monmaney, T. "Remedy's U.S. Sales Zoom, but Quality Control Lags. St. John's Wort: Regulatory Vacuum Leaves Doubt About Potency, Effects of Herb Used for Depression." Los Angeles, CA: *Los Angeles Times*, August 31, 1998.

7. Duke, J. *The Green Pharmacy*. Emmaus, PA: Rodale Press, 1997.

8. American Psychiatric Association. *Diagnostic and Statistical Manual of Mental Disorders. 4th ed.* Washington, DC: American Psychiatric Association, 1995.

9. National Institute of Mental Health. "General Facts About Depression," Bethesda, MD: National Institute of Mental Health, 1997.

10. Medical Economics Company. *Physician's Desk Reference 1998. 52nd ed.* Montvale, NJ: Medical Economics Company, 1997.

11. Kincheloe, L. "Herbal Medicines Can Reduce Costs in HMO." Herbalgram. *The Journal of the American Botanical Council and the Herb Research Foundation*. 1997. (41):49-53.

12. Woelk, H., Burkard, G., and Grunwald, J. "Benefits and Risks of the Hypericum Extract LI 160: Drug Monitoring Study With 3,250 Patients." *Journal of Geriatric Psychiatry and Neurology*. 1994. 7(Supplement 1):S34-8.

13. Laakmann, G., Schule, C., Baghai, T., and Kieser, M. "St. John's Wort in Mild to Moderate Depression: The Relevance of Hyperforin for the Clinical Efficacy." *Pharmacopsychiatry*. June, 1998. 31(Supplement):54-9.

14. Rezvani, A.H. *1998 Annual Meeting of the Research Society on Alcoholism*. Hilton Head, SC: Research Society on Alcoholism, June 23, 1998.

15. Andrews, E. "In Germany, Humble Herb Is Rival to Prozac." New York, NY: *New York Times*, September 9, 1997.

16. Perovic, S. and Muller, W.E.G. "Pharmacological Profile of Hypericum Extract. Effect of Serotonin Uptake by Postsynaptic Receptors." *Arzneimittel-Forschuns*. 1995. 45:1145-8.

17. Thiele, B., Brink, I., and Ploch, M. "Modulation of Cytokine Expression by Hypericum Extract." *Journal of Geriatric Psychiatry and Neurology*. 1994. 7(Supplement 1):S60-2.

18. Harrer, G., Hubner, W.D., and Podzuweit, H. "Effectiveness and Tolerance of the Hypericum Extract LI 160 Compared to Maprotiline: A Multicenter Double-Blind Study." *Journal of Geriatric Psychiatry and Neurology*. 1994. 7(Supplement 1):S24-8.

19. Harrer, G. and Sommer, H. "Treatment of Mild/Moderate Depressions With Hypericum." *Phytomedicine*. 1994. 1:3-8.

Part 5

If You Need More Information

Chapter 49

Mental Health Resources

Academy for Eating Disorders
6728 Old McLean Village Drive
McLean, VA 22010-3906
Phone: 703-556-9222
Fax: 703-556-8729
Website: http://www.acadeatdis.org

A.I.M.
(Agoraphobic in Motion)
1719 Crooks Rd.
Royal Oak, MI 48067-1305
Hotline: 248-547-0400
Phone: 248-547-0705
E-Mail: anny@ameritech.net

American Academy of Child
and Adolescent Psychiatry
3615 Wisconsin Avenue, N.W.
Washington, DC 20016
Phone: 202-966-7300
Fax: 202-966-2891
Website: http://www.aacap.org

American Association of
Suicidology (AAS)
4201 Connecticut Avenue, N.W.,
Suite 408
Washington, DC 20008
Phone: 202-237-2280
Fax: 202-237-2282
Website:
http://www.suicidology.org

American Counseling
Association
5999 Stevenson Ave.
Alexandria, VA 22304
Phone: 703-823-9800
Fax: 703-823-0253
Website:
http://www.counseling.org

Information in this chapter was compiled from many sources deemed reliable; inclusion does not constitute endorsement. All contact information was verified in April 2001.

American Foundation for Suicide Prevention

120 Wall Street, 22nd Floor
New York, NY 10005
Toll Free: 888-333-AFSP
Phone: 212-363-3500
Fax: 212-363-6237
Website: http://www.afsp.org/
E-Mail: inquiry@afsp.org

American Institute for Cognitive Therapy

136 E. 57th, Suite 1101
New York, NY 10022
Phone: 212-308-2440
Fax: 212-308-3099
Website: http://
www.cognitivetherapynyc.com

The American Psychiatric Association

1400 K St., NW
Washington, DC 20005
Phone: 202-682-6000
Fax: 202-682-6850
Website: http://www.psych.org
E-Mail: apa@psych.org

The American Psychiatric Nurses Association

Colonial Place Three
2107 Wilson Blvd., Suite 300-A
Arlington, VA 22201-3042
Phone: 703-243-2443
Fax: 703-243-3390
Website: http://www.apna.org
E-Mail: info@apna.org

The American Psychological Association

750 First St., NE
Washington, DC 20002
Toll Free: 800-374-2721
Phone: 202-336-5500
Website: http://www.apa.org

Anorexia Nervosa and Related Eating Disorders, Inc. (ANRED)

Website: http://www.anred.com

Anxiety Disorders Association of America (ADAA)

11900 Parklawn Drive, Suite 100
Rockville, MD 20852
Phone: 301-231-9350
Fax: 301-231-7392
Website: http://www.adaa.org
E-Mail: AnxDis@adaa.org

Association for Advancement of Behavior Therapy
305 Seventh Ave.
New York, NY 10001-60008
Phone: 212-647-1890
Fax: 212-647-1865
Website: http://www.aabt.org

Bipolar Network News
c/o Stanley Foundation
5430 Grosvenor Lane, Suite 200
Bethesda, MD 20814
Toll Free: 800-518-7326
Fax: 301-571-0768
Website: http://
www.bipolarnetwork.org
E-Mail: info@bipolarnetwork.org

Body Image Program
Butler Hospital
345 Blackstone Blvd.
Providence, RI 02906
Phone: 401-455-6466
Fax: 401-455-6539
Website: http://www.butler.org/
bdd.html

Borderline Personality Disorder Central
Website: http://BPDCentral.com
E-Mail: BPDCentral@aol.com

Center for Loss and Life Transitions
3735 Broken Bow Road
Fort Collins, CO 80526
Phone: 303-226-6050
Website: http://
www.counselingforloss.com
E-Mail:
questions@counselingforloss.com

Center for Mental Health Services
Knowledge Exchange Network
P.O. Box 42490
Washington, DC 20015
Toll-Free: 800-789-2647
Website: http://
www.mentalhealth.org

Child and Adolescent Bipolar Foundation
1187 Wilmett Avenue, PMB #331
Wilmett, IL 60091
Phone: 847-256-8525
Fax: 847-920-9498
Website: www.bpkids.org
E-Mail: cabf@bpkids.org

The Compassionate Friends
(grief assistance)
National Headquarters
P.O. Box 3696
Oak Brook, IL 60522-3696
Toll Free: 877-969-0010
Phone: 630-990-0010
Fax: 630-990-0246
Website: http://
www.compassionatefriends.org

Debtors Anonymous General Service Office
P.O. Box 920888
Needham, MA 02492-0009
Phone: 781-453-2743
Fax: 781-453-2745
Website: http://
www.debtorsanonymous.org
E-Mail:
new@debtorsanonymous.org

Depression and Related Disorders Association
Meyer 3-181, 550 Bldg.
600 North Wolfe Street
Baltimore, MD 21287-7381
Phone: 410-955-4647
Fax: 410-614-3241
Website: http://www.med.jhu.edu/
drada

Emotions Anonymous
P.O. Box 4245
St. Paul, MN 55104-0245
Phone: 612-647-9712
Fax: 651-647-1593
Website: http://
www.emotionsanonymous.org
E-Mail:
info@EmotionsAnonymous.org

Freedom from Fear
308 Seaview Ave.
Staten Island, NY 10305
Phone: 718-351-1717
Fax: 718-667-8893
Website: http://
www.freedomfromfear.org

International Society for Traumatic Stress Studies
60 Revere Dr., Suite 500
Northbrook, IL 60062
Phone: 847-480-9028
Fax: 847-480-9282
Website: http://www.istss.org
E-Mail: istss@istss.org

Internet Mental Health
601 West Broadway, Suite 902
Vancouver, BC V5Z 4C2
Phone: 604-876-2254
Fax: 604-876-4929
Website: http://
www.mentalhealth.com

Kids Hospital Network

P.O. Box 533
Harwich, MA 02645
Phone: 508-430-7122
Website: http://www.harwich.edu/
bear/index.htm#top
E-Mail: bearkids@harwich.edu

Lithium Information Center

7617 Mineral Point Road
Suite 300
Madison, WI 53717
Phone: 608-827-2470
Fax: 608-827-2479
Website: http://
www.healthtechsys.com/
mimlithium.html
E-Mail: mim@healthtechsys.com

Mental Health Net

CMCH Systems
570 Metro Place North
Dublin, OH 43017
Phone: 614-764-0143
Fax: 614-764-0362
Website: http://
www.mentalhelp.net

National Alliance for the Mentally Ill (NAMI)

2107 Wilson Blvd., Suite 300
Arlington, VA 22201
Toll-Free: 800-950-6264
Fax: 703-524-9094
Website: http://www.nami.org

National Alliance for Research on Schizophrenia and Depression (NARSAD)

60 Cutter Mill Road, Suite 404
Great Neck, NY 10021
Toll Free: 800-829-8289
Phone: 516-829-0091
Fax: 516-487-6930
Website: http://www.narsad.org
E-Mail: info@narsad.org

National Anxiety Foundation

3135 Custer Drive
Lexington, KY 40517-4001
Phone: 606-272-7166
Website: http://lexington-on-
line.com/nafmasthead.html

National Association of Anorexia Nervosa and Associated Disorders

P.O. Box 7
Highland Park, IL 60035
Phone: 847-831-3438
Fax: 847-433-4632
Website: http://www.anad.org

The National Association of Social Workers

750 First St., N.E., Suite 700
Washington, DC 20002
Phone: 202-408-8600
Fax: 202-336-8310
Website: http://
www.socialworkers.org

National Crisis Helpline
Toll Free: 800-999-9999

National Depressive and Manic-Depressive Association
730 N. Franklin St., Suite 501
Chicago, Il 60610
Toll Free: 800-826-3632
Phone: 312-642-0049
Fax: 312-642-7243
Website: http://www.ndmda.org

National Domestic Violence Hotline
Toll Free: 800-799-SAFE (7233)

National Eating Disorders Association
(formerly: American Anorexia/ Bulimia Association, Inc.)
603 Stewart Street, Suite 803
Seattle, WA 98101
Phone: 206-382-3587
Internet: http://www.edap.org

National Eating Disorders Organization
6655 South Yale Avenue
Tulsa, OK 74136
Phone: 918-481-4044
Fax: 918-481-4076
Website: http:// www.kidsource.com/nedo

National Foundation for Depressive Illness
P.O. Box 2257
New York, NY 10116
Toll-Free: 800-239-1265
Phone: 212-268-4260
Website: http://www.depression.org

National Hospital for Kids in Crisis
5300 KidsPeace Dr.
Orefield, PA 18069
Toll-Free: 800-446-9543
Fax: 610-799-8801
Website: http://www.kidspeace.org

National Institute of Mental Health
6001 Executive Boulevard, Rm. 8184, MSC 9663
Rockville, MD 20892-9663
Toll-free 800-64-PANIC (647-2642)
Website: http://www.nimh.nih.gov

National Mental Health Association
1021 Prince St.
Alexandria, VA 22314-2971
Toll-Free: 800-969-6642
Website: http://www.nmha.org

National Mental Health Consumers' Self-Help Clearinghouse

1211 Chestnut Street, Suite 1207
Philadelphia, PA 19107
Toll-Free: 800-533-4539
Phone: 215-751-1810
Fax: 215-636-6312
Website: http://
www.mhselfhelp.org
E-Mail: info@mhselfhelp.org

National Organization for Victim Assistance

1730 Park Road, NW
Washington, DC 20010
Toll-Free: 800-TRY-NOVA (879-6682)
Fax: 202-462-2255
Website: http://www.try-nova.org

National Resource Center on Domestic Violence

6400 Flank Dr., Suite 1300
Harrisburg, PA 17112
Toll-Free: 800-537-2238
Fax: 717-545-9456
Website: http://www.ncadv.org

Obsessive Compulsive Disorder Resource Center

Website: www.ocdresource.com

The Obsessive Compulsive Foundation, Inc.

337 Notch Hill Road
North Branford, CT 06471
Phone: 203-315-2190
Fax: 203-315-2196
Website: http://
www.ocfoundation.org
E-Mail: info@ocfoundation.org

Obsessive Compulsive and Spectrum Disorders Association

18653 Ventura Blvd., Suite 414
Tarzana, CA 91356-4174
Phone: 818-990-4830
Fax: 818-760-3784
Website: http://www.ocdhelp.org
E-Mail: admin@ocdhelp.org

Phobics Anonymous

P.O. Box 1180
Palm Springs, CA 92263
Phone: 760-322-COPE (2673)

Rainbows

(grief for death or divorce)
2100 Golf Road, #370
Rolling Meadows, IL 60008-4231
Toll Free: 800-266-3206
Phone: 847-952-1770
Fax: 847-952-1774
Website: http://www.rainbows.org
E-Mail: info@rainbows.org

Rape, Abuse, and Incest National Network
1129 State A6 & A7
Santa Barbara, CA 93101
Toll Free: 800-656-HOPE (4673)
Website: http://www.rain.org

The Samaritans
P.O. Box 1259
Madison Square Station
New York, NY 10159
Suicide Hotline: 212-673-3000
24-hour e-mail service: http://
www.befrienders.org/email.html

SPAN (Suicide Prevention Advocacy Network)
5034 Odin's Way
Marietta, GA 30068
Toll Free: 888-649-1366
Fax: 770-642-1419
Website: http://www.spanusa.org
E-Mail: act@spanusa.org

Suicide Awareness\Voices of Education (SA\VE)
P.O. Box 24507
Minneapolis, MN 55424-0507
Phone: 952-946-7998
Website: http://www.save.org
E-Mail: save@winternet.com

Suicide Information and Education Centre
#201 1615 10th Avenue, SW
Calgary, Alberta T3C 0J7
Phone: 403-245-3900
Fax: 403-245-0299
Website: http://www.siec.ca
E-Mail: siec@suicideinfo.ca

Teen Age Grief, Inc.
P.O. Box 220034
Newhall, CA 91322-0034
Phone: 661-253-1932
Fax: 661-245-2536
Website: http://www.smartlink.net/
~tag
E-Mail: tag@thevine.net

Trichotillomania Learning Center
1215 Mission Street, Suite 2
Santa Cruz, CA 95060
Phone: 831-457-1004
Fax: 831-426-4383

Yellow Ribbon Suicide Prevention Program
P.O. Box 644
Westminster, CO 80030-0644
Phone: 303-429-3530
Fax: 303-426-4496
Website: http://
www.yellowribbon.org
E-Mail:
ask4help@yellowribbon.org

Chapter 50

Resources For Alcoholism And Substance Abuse

12 Step Cyber Cafe
Website: http://www.12steps.org
E-Mail: amark@12steps.org

Addiction Research Foundation
(formerly: Centre for Addiction and Mental Health)
33 Russell Street
Toronto,Ontario M5S 2S1
Toll Free; 800-463-6273
Phone: 535-8501
Website: http://www.camh.net

African American Family Services (AAFS)
2616 Nicollet Ave.
Minneapolis, MN 55408
Toll Free: 800-557-2180
Phone: 612-871-7878
Website: http://www.aafs-mn.org

Al-Anon Family Groups
1600 Corporate Landing Parkway
Virginia Beach, VA 23454-5617
Toll Free: 800-356-9996
Phone: 757-563-1600
Fax: 757-563-1655
Website: http://www.al-anon.org
E-Mail: WSO@al-anon.org

Information in this chapter was compiled from many sources deemed accurate; inclusion does not constitute endorsement. All contact information was verified in April 2001.

Alcoholics Anonymous

P.O. Box 459, Grand Central
Station
New York, NY 10163
Phone: 212-870-3400
Website: http://www.alcoholics-
anonymous.org

America Cares, Inc.

(formerly Drug Free Kids:
America's Challenge)
P.O. Box 60865
Washington, DC 20039
Phone: 301-681-7861
Fax: 301-681-7861
Website: http://
www.ourdrugfreekids.com
E-Mail: info@drugfreekids.org

American Academy of Child and Adolescent Psychiatry

3615 Wisconsin Avenue, N.W.
Washington, DC 20016
Phone: 202-966-7300
Fax: 202-966-2891
Website: http://www.aacap.org

American Council for Drug Education

164 W. 74th St.
New York, NY 10023
Toll Free: 800-488-DRUG (3784)
Website: http://www.acde.org

Center for Substance Abuse Prevention (CSAP)

5600 Fishers Lane, Rockwall II
Rockville, MD 20857
Phone: 301-443-0365
Fax: 301-443-5447
Website: http://www.samhsa.gov/
csap

Center for Substance Abuse Treatment (CSAT)

P.O. Box 2345
Rockville, MD 20847-2345
Toll Free: 800-662-HELP (4357)
Website: http://www.samhsa.gov/
csat

Cocaine Anonymous World Services, Inc.

3740 Overland Avenue, Suite C
Los Angeles, CA 90034
Phone: 310-559-5833
Fax: 310-599-2554
Website: http://www.ca.org
E-Mail: publicinfo@ca.org

Common Sense

Website: http://www.pta.org/
commonsense
E-Mail: info@pta.org

Community Anti-Drug Coalitions of American (CADCA)

901 North Pitt St., Suite 300
Alexandria, VA 22314
Toll Free: 800-54-CADCA
Phone: 703-706-0560
Fax: 703-706-0565
Website: www.cadca.org
E-Mail: info@cadca.org

Connecticut Clearinghouse

334 Farmington Avenue
Plainville, CT 06062
Phone: 800-232-4424
Fax: 860-793-9813
Website: http://ctclearinghouse.org
E-Mail: info@ctclearinghouse.org

Dual Recovery Anonymous

Service Office
P.O. Box 218232
Nashville, TN 37221-8232
Phone: 888-869-9239
Website: http://draonline.org

Families Anonymous

P.O. Box 3475
Culver City, CA 90231
Toll Free: 800-736-9805
Phone: 310-815-8010
Fax: 310-815-9682
Website: http://familiesanonymous.org
E-Mail:
famanon@familiesanonymous.org

Hazelden Foundation

P.O. Box 11
Center City, MN 55012-1011
Toll Free: 800-257-7810
Website: http://www.hazelden.org
E-Mail: info@hazelden.org

Indiana Prevention Resource Center

Indiana University
Creative Arts Building
2735 E. 10th St., Rm. 110
Bloomington, IN 47408-2607
Website: http://
www.drugs.indiana.edu

JACS (Jewish Alcoholics, Chemically Dependent Persons, and Significant Others)

850 7th Avenue
New York, NY 10019
Phone: 212-397-4197
Fax: 212-489-6229
Website: http://www.jacsweb.org
E-Mail: jacs@jacsweb.org

Join Together

441 Stuart St., 7th Fl.
Boston, MA 02116
Phone: 617-437-1500
Fax: 617-437-9394
Website: http://
www.jointogether.org
E-Mail: info@jointogether.org

Marijuana Anonymous World Services
P.O. Box 2912
Van Nuys, CA 91404
Toll Free: 800-766-6779
Website: http://www.marijuana-anonymous.org
E-Mail: office@marijuana-anonymous.org

Moderation Management Network, Inc.
P.O. Box 3055
Point Pleasant, NJ 08742
Phone: 732-295-0940
Website: http://www.moderation.org
E-Mail: moderation@moderation.org

Mothers Against Drunk Driving
511 E. John Carpenter Fwy..
Suite 700
Irving, TX 75062
Toll Free: 800-GET-MADD(438-6233)
Fax: 972-869-2206
Website: http://www.madd.org

Nar-Anon World Service Office
P.O. Box 2562
Palos Verdes Peninsula, CA 90274
Phone: 310-547-5800
Website: http://naranon.com

Narcotics Anonymous
P.O. Box 9999
Van Nuys, CA 91409
Phone: 818-773-9999
Fax: 818-700-0700
Website: http://www.na.org
E-Mail: info@na.org

National Asian Pacific American Families Against Substance Abuse, Inc.
340 E. 2nd Street, Suite 409
Los Angeles, CA 90012
Phone: 213-625-5795
Fax: 213-625-5796
Website: http://www.napafasa.org
E-Mail: napafasa@apanet.org

National Association of Addiction Treatment Providers
501 Randolph Drive
Lititz, PA 17543
Phone: 717-581-1901
Fax:717-581-1902
Website: http://www.naatp.org

National Association for Children of Alcoholics
11426 Rockville Pike, Suite 100
Rockville, MD 20852
Toll Free: 888-554-2627
Phone: 301-468-0985
Website: http://www.health.org/nacoa

National Association for Native American Children of Alcoholics
1402 Third Avenue, Suite 110
Seattle, WA 98101
Toll Free: 800-322-5601
Phone: 206-467-7678
Fax: 206-467-7689
E-Mail: nanacoa@aol.com

National Association of State Alcohol and Drug Abuse Directors
808 17ᵗʰ Street, Suite 410
Washington, DC 20006
Phone: 202-293-0090
Fax: 202-293-1250
Website: http://nasadad.org
E-Mail: dcoffice@nasadad.org

National Clearinghouse for Alcohol and Drug Information
P.O. Box 2345
Rockville, MD 20847-2345
Toll Free: 800-SAY-NOTO (729-6686)
Phone: 301-468-2600
Fax: 301-468-6433
Website: http://www.health.org
E-Mail: info@health.org

National Council on Alcoholism and Drug Dependence, Inc.
20 Exchange Place, Suite 2902
New York, NY 10005
Toll Free: 800-NCA-CALL (622-2255)
Phone: 212-269-7797
Fax: 212-269-7510
Website: http://www.ncadd.org
E-Mail: national@ncadd.org

National Families in Action
2957 Clairmont Road, Suite 150
Atlanta, GA 30329
Phone: 404-248-9676
Fax: 404-246-1312
Website: http://www.emory.edu/NFIA

National Family Partnership
2490 Coral Way
Miami, FL 33145
Toll Free: 800-705-8997
Phone: 305-856-4886
Fax: 305-856-4815
Website: http://www.nfp.org

National Hispano/Latino Community Prevention Network
P.O. Box 2215
Espanola, NM 87532
Phone: 505-747-1889
Fax: 505-747-1623
E-Mail: hacc@la-tierra.com

National Inhalant Prevention Coalition
2904 Kerbey Lane
Austin, TX 78703
Toll Free: 800-269-4237
Phone: 512-480-8953
Fax: 512-477-3932
Website: http://www.inhalants.org
E-Mail: nipc@io.com

National Institute on Drug Abuse
6001 Executive Blvd., Room 5213
Bethesda, MD 20892-9561
Phone: 301-443-1124
Website: http://www.nida.nih.gov
E-Mail:
information@lists.nida.nih.gov

Online Recovery
Website: http://onlinerecovery.org

Parents and Adolescents Recovering Together Successfully (PARTS)
7825 Engineer Road, Suite 202
San Diego, CA 92111
Phone: 858-292-TEEN (8336)
Fax: 858-560-5445
Website: http://
www.teendrughelp.org

Partnership for a Drug-Free America
405 Lexington Ave., 16th Floor
New York, NY 10174
Phone: 212-922-1560
Fax: 212-922-1570
Website: http://
www.drugfreeamerica.org

Rational Recovery Systems, Inc.
P.O. Box 800
Lotus, CA 95651-0800
Phone: 530-621-4374
Fax: 530-622-4296
Website: http://www.rational.org
E-Mail: home@rational.org

Research Institute on Addiction
1021 Main Street
Buffalo, NY 14203
Phone: 716-887-2566
Fax: 716-887-2252
Website: http://www.ria.buffalo.edu

Safe and Drug-Free Schools Program
U.S. Department of Education
400 Maryland Ave. SW
Washington, DC 20202-6123
Toll Free: 877-433-7827 for publications
Phone: 202-260-3954
Website: http://www.ed.gov/
offices/OESE/SDFS

SMART Recovery
7537 Mentor Avenue, Suite 306
Mentor, OH 44060
Phone: 440-951-5357
Fax: 440-951-5358
Website: http://
www.smartrecovery.org
E-Mail: srmail1@aol.com

Women for Sobriety, Inc.
P.O. Box 618
Quakertown, PA 18951
Phone: 215-536-8026
Fax: 215-538-9026
Website: http://
www.womenforsobriety.org

Index

Index

Page numbers that appear in *Italics* refer to illustrations. Page numbers that have a small 'n' after the page number refer to information shown as Notes at the beginning of each chapter. Page numbers that appear in **Bold** refer to information contained in boxes on that page (except Notes information at the beginning of each chapter).

A

AAFS *see* African American Family Services

AAS *see* American Association of Suicidology

"About Early-Onset Bipolar Disorder" (CABF) 127n

Academy for Eating Disorders, contact information **246**, 373

acarophobia **194**

acousticophobia **194**

acquaintance rape *see* date rape

acquired immune deficiency syndrome (AIDS) 12

acrophobia 152, **194**, 196

active listening 29–30, **30**
see also communication skills

acute stress disorder 154–55, 174

ADAA *see* Anxiety Disorders Association of America

Adapin (doxepin) 170

ADD *see* attention deficit disorder

Adderall (dextroamphetamine) 238

addiction, bipolar disorder 131

The Addiction Letter (Manisses Communications Group) 293n

Addiction Research Foundation, contact information 381

ADHD *see* attention deficit hyperactivity disorder

adrenaline 35

advocacy, defined **344**

advocacy groups 343–52

affect, defined **230**

affective disorder, defined **118**

African American Family Services (AAFS), contact information 381

age factor
anxiety disorders 158–59
self-injury 254

agoraphobia
body dysmorphic disorder **250**
defined **194**, 196
described 151, 201–2
treatment 168, 170

Agoraphobic in Motion (A.I.M.), contact information 373

aichmophobia **194**

AIDS *see* acquired immune deficiency syndrome

ailurophobia **194**

A.I.M. *see* Agoraphobic in Motion

Al-Anon Family Groups, contact information 381

Alcoholics Anonymous, contact information 382

alcoholism
  anxiety disorders 162, 166
  resource information 381–87
alcohol use
  grief 86
  personal pressures 61–63
  social phobia 199
  violence 66
algophobia **194**
alprazolam 171, 197, **198**
amaxophobia **194**
America Cares, Inc., contact information 382
American Academy of Child and Adolescent Psychiatry, contact information 125, 291, 373, 382
American Anorexia/Bulimia Association, Inc. *see* National Eating Disorders Association
American Association of Suicidology (AAS), contact information 124, 291, 373
American Council for Drug Education, contact information 382
American Counseling Association, contact information 373
American Foundation for Suicide Prevention, contact information 291, 374
American Institute for Cognitive Therapy, contact information 374
American Psychiatric Association (APA)
  contact information 191, **332**, 374
  depression statistics 108–9, **116**
  eating disorders 21
  publications
    controlling anger 35n
    love and violent behavior 55n
    panic disorder 181n
    psychotherapy 337n
The American Psychiatric Nurses Association, contact information 374
American Psychological Association (APA)
  contact information **332**, 374
  described 190–91
  publications 181n, 337n
amygdala 156
anabolic steroids 21
Anafranil (clomipramine) 170, 221, 251
androphobia **194**

anger
  causes 36, 38
  control 37–38, 39–43, **42**, **44**
  described 35–36
  expressing anger 36–37
  grief 86–87
  treatment 44
  triggers 39
anger management 37
animal phobias 196
anorexia nervosa
  defined **18**, **244**
  described 242
  statistics 21, 103
  symptoms **242**
Anorexia Nervosa and Related Disorders, Inc. (ANRED), contact information **246**, 374
ANRED *see* Anorexia Nervosa and Related Disorders, Inc.
"Answers to Your Questions about Panic Disorder" (APA) 181n
anthropophobia **194**
anti-anxiety medications 141, 189, 197, 200
anti-convulsive medications, bipolar disorder 136, 359
antidepressant medications
  anxiety disorders treatment 167–72
  attention deficit disorder 238
  defined **364**
  described 112–14
  panic disorder 189
  post-traumatic stress disorder 216
  social phobia 200, 207, 210
  suicides 288
  types 108, 355–56
antipsychotic medications 141, 279–80, 359–60
antisocial personality disorder 230
anxiety
  defined **148**, **178**, **186**
  symptoms 149–50
Anxiety, Phobias, and Panic (Peurifoy) **185**
anxiety disorders
  causes 155–58
  defined **148**
  described 101, 147–76
  diagnosis 163–66, **164**
  generalized, described 101
  risk factors 158–63

anxiety disorders, continued
  symptoms 149–55
  treatment *167*, 167–76, 360–62
Anxiety Disorders Association of America
  (ADAA) 353n
  contact information 362, 374
Anxiety Disorders Interview Schedule 166
anxiolytics, defined **178**
APA *see* American Psychiatric Association;
  American Psychological Association
apiphobia **194**
arachnophobia **194**, 196
arousal, defined **148**
art therapy **330**
assertiveness training 44
Association for Advancement of Behavior
  Therapy, contact information 375
astraphobia **194**
atenolol 172, 197, **198**
Ativan (lorazepam) 141, 171
attention deficit disorder (ADD) 156, 235–40
attention deficit hyperactivity disorder
  (ADHD) 4
  bipolar disorder 123–24, 128, 134
  defined **128**, **236**
  described 102
attention intervention 175
autism spectrum disorder, described 103
avoidant personality disorder 230
azapirones 171–72, 360

B

Barr, Brian 303n, 306
basal-ganglia thalamocortical pathway 156
bathophobia **194**
BDD *see* body dysmorphic disorder
Beck Anxiety Inventory 166
behavior therapy
  defined **178**
  described **330**
  obsessive-compulsive disorder 221–22
  panic disorder **186**
  phobias 200
  self-injury 259–63
  social phobia 212
  see also cognitive behavioral therapy; cog-
    nitive therapy

benzodiazepines
  anxiety disorders 168, 360–61
  defined **178**
  described 170–71
  phobias 197, 210
bereavement, defined **84**
beta blockers 172, 197, 200, 210, 361
binge eating disorder
  defined **18**, **244**
  described 243
  symptoms **243**
bipolar depression 109
bipolar disorder 4
  defined **122**
  described 102, 121
  diagnosis 133–37
  early-onset 127–46
  mood swings 102
  resource information 124–25
  symptoms **102**, 121–25, 129–31, **132**
  treatment 124, 137–43, 357–59
Bipolar Network News, contact information 375
bisexual adolescents, personal pressures 61
body dysmorphic disorder (BDD) 247–
  52
"Body Dysmorphic Disorder (BDD) and
  Body Image Program" 247n
body image
  media 19–20
  negative body image 17–18, **20**
  see also dieting; self-esteem
Body Image Program, contact information
  251, 375
  see also Butler Hospital
body piercings **254**
borderline personality disorder
  bipolar disorder 134
  described 231
Borderline Personality Disorder Central,
  contact information 375
boxing 19
breathing retraining, anxiety disorders 175
bromidrosiphobia **194**
brontophobia **194**
*The Brown University Child and Adolescent
  Behavior Letter* 297n, 303n
bulimia nervosa 21
  defined **18**, **244**

bulimia nervosa, continued
    described 103, 242–43
    symptoms **243**
bulking up, body image 21
bupropion 108
BuSpar (buspirone) 141, 171–72
buspirone 171–72, 179
Butler Hospital (Providence, RI) 247n, **251**
    see also Body Image Program

C

CABF *see* Child and Adolescent Bipolar
    Foundation
CADCA *see* Community Anti-Drug Coa-
    litions of America
calcium channel blockers 141
Call to Action to Prevent Suicide (Satcher)
    286
Capgras syndrome **268**, 271–72, 273
carbamazepine 140, 358
Carey, Drew 115
catatonic schizophrenia 278
Celexa (citalopram) 168, 251
The Center for Environmental Therapeu-
    tics (CET), contact information 119
Center for Loss and Life Transitions, con-
    tact information 375
Center for Mental Health Services
    (CMHS)
    contact information **332**, 375
    publications 99n, 104
Center for Substance Abuse Prevention
    (CSAP), contact information 382
Center for Substance Abuse Treatment
    (CSAT), contact information 382
CET *see* The Center for Environmental
    Therapeutics
chemical hypersensitivity, anxiety disorders
    157
child abuse
    defined **70**
    described 69–70
    grief 84
    treatment 71, 169
Child and Adolescent Bipolar Foundation
    (CABF) 127n
    contact information **144**, 375

child neglect, defined **70**
Children's Hospital for Teens (Akron, OH)
    15, 29n, 31n, 51n, 69n, 335n
"Children's Mental Health: Bipolar Disor-
    der" (NMHA) 121n
chlordiazepoxide 171
chronic grief, defined **84**
chronophobia **194**
cimetidine 171
citalopram 168, 251
claustrophobia 152, **194**, 196
Clerembault's syndrome 267
clomipramine 170, 251
clonazepam 171
clonidine 172
CMHS *see* Center for Mental Health Ser-
    vices
Cocaine Anonymous World Services, Inc.,
    contact information 382
cognition, defined **298**
cognitive behavioral therapy
    anxiety disorders treatment 167, 172–75
    body dysmorphic disorder 251
    computer addiction 226
    eating disorders 146
    social phobia 210–11
    see also behavior therapy; cognitive
        therapy
"Cognitive characteristics predict adoles-
    cent suicide attempts" (Spirito) 297n
cognitive restructuring, anger control 40–41
cognitive therapy
    defined **178**
    described **330**
    panic disorder 188
    suicide prevention 300–301
    see also behavior therapy; cognitive be-
        havioral therapy
coitophobia **194**
Columbia University
    contact information 119
    publications 117n
commitments 53
Common Sense website 382
communication skills 29–30, **32**
    anger 38
    anger control 41–42
    self-injury 265
    see also active listening

Community Anti-Drug Coalitions of America (CADCA), contact information 383

The Compassionate Friends, contact information 376

compulsion, defined **148, 222**

compulsive eating 21

computer addiction 225–27

"Computer Addiction: Is It Real or Virtual?" (Harvard Mental Health Letter) 225n

conduct disorder 4
    bipolar disorder **123**, 134
    described 102–3

Connecticut Clearinghouse, contact information 383

control delusion **268**

"Controlling Anger—Before It Controls You" (APA) 35n

Cooke, David A. 253n

coprophobia **194**

Cotard's syndrome 272

counseling
    anger 44
    child abuse 71
    divorce **81**
    eating disorders 246
    schizophrenia 280
    stress 49
    suicidal behavior 313
    violence 66

Cowdry, Rex 285n

CSAP see Center for Substance Abuse Prevention

CSAT see Center for Substance Abuse Treatment

cultural beliefs, personal pressures 61

Cunningham, Linda 83n

cyclothymia 130

cynophobia **194**, 196

D

date rape 56, 58, **62**

dating
    grief 84
    rules 59

"Dealing with the Depths of Depression" (Nordenberg) 107n

Debtors Anonymous General Service Office, contact information 376

Deffenbacher, Jerry 38, 43

delinquency, bipolar disorder **123**

delusional disorders 267–74
    see also *individual disorders*

delusions
    defined **268**
    described 269–70
    of grandeur **230**, 267–68, **270**

"Delusions and Delusional Disorders" (Harvard Mental Health Letter) 267n

Depakote (valproic acid) 140, 358

dependent personality disorder 231

depression
    anxiety disorders 160–61, 166, 179
    bipolar disorder **123**, 134
    body dysmorphic disorder **250**
    defined **122, 128**
    described 4, 25, 27, 101–2
    eating disorders 245
    hopelessness 298–99
    obsessive-compulsive disorder 220
    seasonal affective disorder 117
    social phobia 199
    statistics **108**
    substance abuse 293–95
    symptoms **26**, 130
    treatment 107–16, 200, 353–60, 364–67
    see also *individual types*

Depression and Related Disorders Association
    contact information 362, 376
    publications 353n

"Depression and substance use can be a lethal combination for teens" (The Addiction Letter) 293n

dermatrophobia **194**

Dexedrine (dextroamphetamine) 238

dextroamphetamine 238

dextrophobia **194**

DHHS see US Department of Health and Human Services

Diagnostic and Statistical Manual (DSM)
    bipolar disorder **128**, 133
    depressive disorder 111
    personality disorders 229, **230**
    self-injury **256**, 257

diazepam 171, 197, **198**

dieting 21
diet pills 21
disabilities, personal pressures 61
discontinuation syndrome, described **359**
disorganized schizophrenia 278
dissociation
  defined **256**
  self-injury 263–64
divalproex sodium 140
divorce 73–81
  grief 84
"Divorce and the American Family"
  (Dreher) 73n
domestic violence, personal pressures 60–
  61
dopamine, defined **354**
doxepin 170
Dreher, Nancy 73n, 235n
drug abuse
  bipolar disorder **123**
  grief 86
  personal pressures 61–63
  violence 66
  see also substance abuse
Dual Recovery Anonymous, contact information 383
dysfunctional grief, defined **84**
dysmorphic, defined **248**
dysthymia 109

E

eating disorders 4
  defined **18**
  described 21, 103, 241–46
  self-esteem 22
  self-injury 254
ECT *see* electroconvulsive therapy
Effexor (venlafaxine) 108, 112, 169, 357
efficacy, defined **354**
Elavil 356
electroconvulsive therapy (ECT)
  bipolar disorder 142
  described 113–14, **330**
emotional abuse 55–68, **62**, 69–71
emotions
  defined **52**, **230**
  difficulties 90

emotions, continued
  divorce 76–78
  see also feelings; *individual emotions or
    feelings*
Emotions Anonymous, contact information 376
empathy, defined **230**
energy hormones 35
environmental factors, depression 110
equinophobia 196
eremophobia **194**
ergasiophobia **194**
erotomania
  defined **268**
  described 267, **270**
erythrophobia **194**
Eskalith (lithium) 140
esteem *see* self-esteem
exercise, depression 114
exposure and response prevention 221–22

F

Families Anonymous, contact information
  383
family issues
  anxiety disorders 156–57
  bipolar disorder 131–32
  divorce 73–81
  mental disorders 99
  mental illness
    parents 89–92
    siblings 93–96
  stress 46
Family Service America (Milwaukee, WI)
  74, **78**
family therapy **330**
feelings
  anger 35–44
  sadness 25–28, **26**
  self-esteem 11–16
  self-injury 262
  see also emotions; *individual emotions or
    feelings*
fenfluramine 21
fen-phen 21
"Fifteen Prevalent Myths Concerning
  Adolescent Suicide" (King) 307n

"Fighting Phobias: The Things That Go Bump In The Mind" (Hall) 193n
financial concerns
    divorce 79–80
    support groups 333–34
5-HT2 blocker 169
fluoxetine 108, 168, **198**, 200, 251
fluvoxamine 168, 169, **198**, 200, 251
Focus Adolescent Services 229n
forced sex *see* date rape
Freedom from Fear, contact information 376
Fregoli delusion 272
friends
    chosing **14–15**
    violence 66–67
    see also peer pressure; relationships

G

gabapentin 140, 359
Gabitrol (tiagabine) 141
GAD *see* generalized anxiety disorder
gamma amino butyric acid receptor modulator 172
gamophobia **194**
Garner, David M. 19
gay adolescents *see* homosexual adolescents
gender factor
    anxiety disorders 159
    attention deficit disorder 235
    body image 18–19
    panic disorder 183
    self-injury 254
    stereotypes 59–60
    suicidal behavior 311
generalized anxiety disorder (GAD)
    age factor 159
    bipolar disorder 134
    defined **148**, **178**
    described 147, 177–79
    symptoms 150
    treatment *167*, 360
genetic factors
    anxiety disorders 156–57
    bipolar disorder 131–32
    depression 110–11
    eating disorders 245

genetic factors, continued
    obsessive-compulsive disorder 216
    personality disorders 233
    schizophrenia 276
    social phobia 206
"Getting Along With Others" (Children's Hospital for Teens) 29n
"Go Ask Alice!: Seasonal Affective Disorder (SAD)" (Columbia University) 117n
Gold, Tracy 21
Goldstein, David M. 353n
grief
    adolescents 83–88
    coping strategies 87–88
    divorce 73
    see also grief reaction
"Grief and the Adolescent" (Cunningham) 83n
grief reaction, defined **84**
group therapy **330**
gynephobia **194**

H

hair pulling *see* trichotillomania
halazepam 171
Hall, Lynne L. 193n
hamartophobia **194**
Hamilton Anxiety Rating Scale 166
haphephobia **194**
harpaxophobia **194**
Harvard Mental Health Letter 225n, 267n
Hazelden Foundation, contact information 383
hedonophobia **194**
Hellander, Martha 127
hemophobia **194**
Henrich, Christy 21
herb, defined **364**
histamine 169
histrionic personality disorder 231
hodophobia **194**
homosexual adolescents
    personal pressures 61
    violent behavior 57
"How to Find Help through Psychotherapy" (APA) 337n

"How to Make Peace with Your Body"
    (Maynard) 17n
"How to Start a Self-Help/Advocacy
    Group" (Rogers) 343n
"How to Stop a Panic Attack" (Rager) **185**
humiliation 55
humor, anger control 42–43
hydrophobia **194**
hylophobia **195**
hypengyophobia **195**
hyperactivity
    defined **236**
    symptoms 237–38
hypertension, defined **36**
hyperventilation 175
hypnophobia **195**
hypochondria, defined **268**
hypomania 130

I

ichthyophobia **195**
IEP individualized education plan
"If You Are Feeling Suicidal" (SIEC) 317n
imagery
    anger control 39
    defined **36**
    stress 49
imipramine 112, 170
impulse-control disorder, defined **226**
Inderal (propranolol) 172, 197, **198**
Indiana Prevention Resource Center, con-
    tact information 383
individualized education plan (IEP), bipo-
    lar disorder 143–44
"Information for Brothers and Sisters of
    People with Neurobiological Disorders"
    (NAMI) 93n
intermittent explosive disorder, bipolar dis-
    order 134
Internet Mental Health, contact informa-
    tion 376
interpersonal therapy 175
iophobia **195**
irrational fear *see* phobias
irritability, defined **122**
irritable bowel syndrome 179
isolation, in relationships 65

isradipine 141
"Is This Love?" (Children's Hospital for
    Teens) 51n

J

JACD *see* Jewish Alcoholics, Chemically
    Dependent Persons, and Significant
    Others
Jackson, Sheryl 196–97
Janimine (imipramine) 170
jealousy 267, **270**
Jewish Alcoholics, Chemically Dependent
    Persons, and Significant Others (JACS),
    contact information 383
Join Together, contact information 383
Journal of School Health 307n

K

keraunophobia **195**
Kids Hospital Network, contact informa-
    tion 377
King, Keith A. 307n, 316
Klonopin (clonazepam) 141, 171

L

lalophobia **195**
Lamictal (lamotrigine) 141, 359
lamotrigine 141
late paraphrenia 269
Laughren, Thomas 108, 109, 112, **113**,
    114, 115, 206
learning disorders, described 102
Lebelle, Linda 229n
lesbian adolescents *see* homosexual adoles-
    cents
levophobia **195**
Librium (chlordiazepoxide) 171
light therapy
    bipolar disorder 142
    seasonal affective disorder 111, 118–19
listening, active **30**
    see also active listening; communication
        skills

lithium
  bipolar disorder 357–58, **359**
  defined **128**
  described 140
Lithium Information Center, contact information 377
Lithobid (lithium) 140
locus ceruleus 155
lorazepam 171
love
  described 51–53
  violent behavior 55–68
"Love Doesn't Have to Hurt Teens" (APA) 55n
Luvox (fluvoxamine) 168, **198**, 200, 221, 251, 357

M

major depression 109, 112
malaise, seasonal affective disorder 117
male privilege abuse 56, **62**
Malignant Self-Love: Narcissism Revisited (Vaknin) 232
mania
  defined **122, 128**
  symptoms 130
manic depressive illness *see* bipolar disorder
MAOI *see* monoamine oxidase inhibitors (MAOI)
Marijuana Anonymous World Services, contact information 384
marriage 52
Marta, Suzy Yehl 76
Maynard, Cindy 17n
McCann, Una 205, 211
meditation 114
"Mental, Emotional, and Behavioral Disorders in Children and Adolescents" (CMHS) 99n
mental health
  checklist **8**
  defined **4**
  described 4–6
  resource information 291–92, 373–80
  therapy options **330**
  treatment guidelines 327–34
  see also mental health problems

"Mental Health and You: A Mental Health Checklist" (NMHA) **6, 8**
Mental Health Net, contact information 377
mental health problems **4**
  causes 4–5, 99
  described **100**
  warning signs 5–7
  see also mental health
mental health professionals 328–31
"Mental Illness in the Family: Part 2—Guidelines for Seeking Care" (NMHA) 327n
Mesta Vista Hospital (San Diego, CA) 18
MET *see* motivational enhancement therapy
methylphenidate 238
mirtazapine 108, 169
misidentification delusions 271–73
mitral valve prolapse 165
MK-869 172
Moderation Management Network, Inc., contact information 384
molysmophobia **195**
monoamine oxidase inhibitors (MAOI) 112, 170, 200, 207, 355–56, 361
mood changes
  bipolar disorder 102
  divorce 77
mood disorders
  described 101–2
  treatment 353–60
mood stabilizers 139, 140–41
Mothers Against Drunk Driving, contact information 384
motivational enhancement therapy (MET) 226–27
movement therapy **330**
music therapy **330**

N

NAMI *see* National Alliance for the Mentally Ill
Nar-Anon World Service Office, contact information 384
narcissistic personality disorder 231
Narcotics Anonymous, contact information 384

Nardil (phenelzine) 112, 170, **198**, 200, 356

NARSAD *see* National Alliance for Research on Schizophrenia and Depression

National Alliance for Research on Schizophrenia and Depression (NARSAD), contact information 116, **281**, 377

National Alliance for the Mentally Ill (NAMI)
contact information 116, **281**, **332**, 377
depression statistics 109, 111
publications 93n, 285n, 321n

National Anxiety Foundation, contact information 377

National Asian Pacific American Families Against Substance Abuse, Inc., contact information 384

National Association for Children of Alcoholics, contact information 384

National Association for Native American Children of Alcoholics, contact information 385

National Association of Addiction Treatment Providers, contact information 384

National Association of Anorexia Nervosa and Associated Disorders, contact information 377

The National Association of Social Workers, contact information 377

National Association of State Alcohol and Drug Abuse Directors, contact information 385

National Center for Complementary and Alternative Medicine (NCCAM)
contact information 368
publications 363n

National Clearinghouse for Alcohol and Drug Information, contact information 385

National Council on Alcoholism and Drug Dependence, Inc., contact information 385

National Crisis Helpline 378

National Depressive and Manic-Depressive Association 109, 115
contact information 116, 378

National Domestic Violence Hotline **68**, 378

National Eating Disorders Association, contact information **246**, 378

National Eating Disorders Organization, contact information **246**, 378

National Families in Action, contact information 385

National Family Partnership, contact information 385

National Foundation for Depressive Illness, contact information 378

National Hispano/Latino Community Prevention Network, contact information 385

National Hospital for Kids in Crisis, contact information **28**, 378

National Inhalant Prevention Coalition, contact information 386

National Institute of Mental Health (NIMH)
contact information **28**, 116, **281**, **332**, 378
publications
generalized anxiety disorder (GAD) 177n

National Institute on Drug Abuse, contact information 386

National Mental Health Association (NMHA)
contact information **28**, 124, **246**, **281**, **332**, 378
publications **6**, **8**, 327n
bipolar disorder 121n
mental health **6**, **8**
mental illness 327n
schizophrenia 275n
self-esteem 11n, 22
stress 45n

National Mental Health Consumers' Self-Help Clearinghouse, contact information 352, 379

National Mental Health Services Knowledge Exchange Network, contact information 9

National Organization for Victim Assistance, contact information **68**, 379

National Resource Center on Domestic Violence, contact information **68**, 379

NCCAM *see* National Center for Complementary and Alternative Medicine

necrophobia **195**

nefazodone 108, 169

Nemours Foundation
publications 25n

Neurontin (gabapentin) 140–41, 359
neurotransmitters
  anxiety disorders 155
  defined **354**
  described 110
  eating disorders 245
  social phobia 199
Nidus Information Services, Inc. 147n
nihilistic delusion **268**
NIMH *see* National Institute of Mental
  Health
nimodipine 141
NMHA *see* National Mental Health Association
noctiphobia **195**
noradrenaline 35
Nordenberg, Liora 107n
Nordenberg, Tamar 203n
norepinephrine
  defined **354**
  depression 110, 114
Norpramin 356
nosophobia **195**
nutritional supplements, bipolar disorder
  142
nyctophobia **195**

O

obsession
  defined **222, 230, 248, 268**
  versus delusion 270–71
Obsessive Compulsive and Spectrum Disorders Association, contact information
  379
"Obsessive-Compulsive Disorder (OCD)"
  (*Clinical Reference Systems*) 219n
obsessive-compulsive disorder (OCD)
  age factor 158–59
  bipolar disorder 134
  body dysmorphic disorder **250**
  defined **148, 222**
  described 101, 147, 219–23, 231
  diagnosis 221
  family influence 157
  rituals **220**
  symptoms 152–53
  treatment *167*, 170, 173–75, 200, 221–23

Obsessive Compulsive Disorder Resource
  Center, contact information 379
The Obsessive Compulsive Foundation,
  Inc., contact information 223, 379
OCD *see* obsessive-compulsive disorder
ochlophobia **195**
odontiatophobia 152, 196–97
ombrophobia **195**
Omega-3 oil (fish oil) 142
Online Recovery website 386
ophidiophobia **195**, 196
oppositional-defiant disorder 134
organic, defined **256**
Orzack, Maressa Hecht 225n
Osmond, Donny 203–5, 211–12, 213
overeating, compulsive 21

P

pagoclone 172
Pamelor 356
panic, defined **148, 186**
panic attacks
  defined **149, 186**
  described 181–82
  treatment *167*, **184–85**
panic disorder
  bipolar disorder 134
  body dysmorphic disorder **250**
  causes 183–86
  defined **186**
  described 101, 181–83
  side effects 187–88
  statistics **182**
  symptoms 150–51
  treatment 168, 170, **184–85**, 188–90
panphobia **195**
Papolos, Demitri 127
paralipophobia **195**
paranoid personality disorder 231
paranoid schizophrenia 278
paraphrenia, late 269
parasitophobia **195**
Parents and Adolescents Recovering Together Successfully (PARTS), contact information 386
Parnate (tranylcypromine) 170, **198**, 200,
  356

paroxetine 108, 168, **198**, 200, 204, 251
paroxysmal supraventricular tachycardia
  165
Partnership for a Drug-Free America, contact information 386
PARTS *see* Parents and Adolescents Recovering Together Successfully
pathological, defined **36**
pathophobia **195**
Paxil (paroxetine) 108, 112, 168, **198**, 200,
  201, 204, 207, 210, 212, 221, 251, 357
Paxipam (halazepam) 171
peer pressure
  described 31–34
  self-esteem 12
  stress 46
  see also friends; relationships
"Peer Pressure" (Children's Hospital for
  Teens) 31n
peniaphobia **195**
performance anxiety 151–52, 167
persecution delusion **268, 270**
personality disorders 229–33
  see also *individual disorders*
"Pete's Story" (Dreher) 235n
Peurifoy, Reneau **185**
phagophobia **195**
"Pharmacological Treatment of Mood Disorders" (Goldstein) 353n
pharmacophobia **195**
phasmophobia **195**
phenelzine 112, 170, **198**, 200
phobias 193–202
  defined **149**
  described 101, 152
  family influence 157
  treatment *167*, 197–98
  see also *individual phobias*
phobic disorders, symptoms 151–52
Phobics Anonymous, contact information
  379
phobophobia **195**
photophobia **195**
physical abuse 55–68, **62**, 69–71
"Physical and Emotional Abuse"
  (Children's Hospital for Teens) 69n
physiological, defined **36**
piercings *see* body piercings
pnigophobia **195**

Pomice, Eva 19
Pondimin 21
post-traumatic stress disorder (PTSD) 85,
  148
  bipolar disorder 134
  defined **149, 216**
  described 101, 215–16
  diagnosis 163
  outlook 162–63
  risk factors 160
  statistics **215**
  symptoms 153–55
  treatment 169, 173–75, 216–17
potamophobia **195**
pregnancy, personal pressures 61
problem-solving, anger control 41
progressive muscle relaxation, defined **178**
propranolol 172, 197, **198**
Prozac (fluoxetine) 108, 112, 113, 168, **198**,
  200, 221, 251, 356
psychoanalysis 175
  defined **330, 338**
psychological abuse **62**
psychologists, defined **338**
psychology, defined **338**
Psychology Today
  body image survey 20
psychopathology, defined **298, 338**
psychopharmacology, defined **338, 354**
psychosis, defined **268**
psychotherapy
  anxiety disorders treatment 175
  bipolar disorder 142
  defined **122, 338**
  depression 114
  eating disorders 246
  mental health care 337–41
  post-traumatic stress disorder 216
psychotic, defined **256, 354**
psychotropic drugs, defined **338, 354**
pterygophobia 152, 196
PTSD *see* post-traumatic stress disorder
pyrophobia **195**

Q

"QPR, Ask a Question, Save a Life"
  (Quinnett) 321n

"Quick Facts About Generalized Anxiety
   Disorder" (NIMH) 177n
Quinnett, Paul 321n

R

Rager, Karen **185**
Rainbows
   contact information 379
   described 76, **78**
Rape, Abuse, and Incest National Network,
   contact information **68**, 380
rape, statutory 63
   see also date rape
Rappaport, Mary 108, 115
Rational Recovery Systems, Inc., contact
   information 386
reactive attachment disorder, bipolar disorder 134
reduplicative paramnesia 272
Redux 21
relationships
   described 29–30
   difficulties 89–90
   mature love 51–53
   sadness 27
   sexual 52
   see also friends; peer pressur
relaxation, defined **36**
relaxation therapy
   anger control 39
   anxiety disorders treatment 175
   panic disorder 189
   stress 48
Remeron (mirtazapine) 108, 112, 169, 356
remission, defined **277**
Research Institute on Addiction, contact
   information 386
residual schizophrenia 278–79
Risperdal 141
Ritalin (methylphenidate) 238
rituals
   defined **256**
   self-injury 260
Rogers, Joseph A. 343n
role models **32**
Ross, Jerilyn 205, 207, 211
routines, stress 47

S

SAD *see* seasonal affective disorder
Safe and Drug-Free Schools Program, contact information 386
St. John's Wort
   bipolar disorder 142
   described **113**, 363–70
"St. John's Wort Fact Sheet" 363n
The Samaritans, contact information 380
same-sex relationships, violent behavior *see*
   homosexual adolescents
Satcher, David 286
SA\VE *see* Suicide Awareness\Voices of
   Education
schizoaffective disorder 279
schizoid personality disorder 231
schizophrenia
   bipolar disorder **123**, 134
   caretakers **278**
   causes 275–76
   defined **277**
   described 103, 275
   statistics **276**
   symptoms 276–78, 279–81
   types 278–79
"Schizophrenia: What You Need to Know"
   (NMHA) 275n
schizotypal personality disorder 231
scopophobia **195**
seasonal affective disorder (SAD)
   defined **118**
   described 110–11, 117–19
selective serotonin reuptake inhibitors
   (SSRI) 113, 167, 168–69, 200, 355–57,
   361
"Self-Esteem" (Children's Hospital for
   Teens) **15**
self-esteem
   body image 22
   described 11–13
   esteem, defined 11
   how to find yourself 14–15
   positive **12**, 16, **16**, 22–24
   sadness 27
   stress 46
self-help groups 343–52
self-image *see* body image

self-injury
  categories 255–57
  communication 264–65
  described 253–54
  treatment 258–63
serious emotional disturbances, described **100**
Seroquel 141
serotonin 110, 206, 288
  defined **354**
  see also selective serotonin reuptake in-
    hibitors
sertraline 108, 168, 169, **198**, 200, 251
Serzone (nefazodone) 108, 112, 169, 357
sexual abuse **62**
sexually transmitted diseases (STD) 12
sexual relations
  anti-depressant medications 169
  date rape 56, 58
  grief 86
  relationships 52
Shaffer, David 285n, 293
shock therapy *see* electroconvulsive therapy
side effect, defined **354, 364**
Sinequan (doxepin) 170
Singer, Mark 81
Sitch, Kathryn 77
Sletten, Chris 200–201
SLTBR *see* The Society for Light Treatment and Biological Rhythms
SMART Recovery, contact information 387
social phobia
  body dysmorphic disorder **250**
  causes 206–7
  defined **149, 204**
  described 199–201, 203–5
  self-test 208–9
  statistics **212**
  symptoms 151–52
  treatment 168, 207, 210–13
"Social Phobias" (Nordenberg) 203n
The Society for Light Treatment and Biological Rhythms (SLTBR), contact information 119
socioeconomic factors
  anxiety disorders 159
  suicidal behavior 313
somatic delusions 268, **268**, **270**
SPAN *see* Suicide Prevention Advocacy
  Network

Spielberger, Charles 35, 37
Spirito, Anthony 297n, 301
sports activities
  body image 18–19
  self-esteem **16**
SSRI *see* selective serotonin reuptake inhibitors
Stanley Foundation, contact information 375
starvation, self-induced *see* anorexia
  nervosa
statutory rape, defined 63
STD *see* sexually transmitted diseases
stereotypes, described 59–60
stress
  bipolar disorder **123**
  generalized anxiety disorder 179
  mental disorders 99
  mental health issues 3
  panic disorder 183
  survival guide 45–49
  symptoms 46
  treatment 47–49
stress disorder, acute 154–55
stress response 147
substance abuse
  anxiety disorders 162, 166, 179
  bipolar disorder 131
  depression 110, 293–95
  post-traumatic stress disorder 163
  resource information 381–87
  self-injury 254
  see also drug abuse
Substance Abuse and Mental Health Services Administration 3n
substance-P 172
suicide
  adolescents 285–92
  anxiety disorders 160–61
  attempted 297–301
  causes 288
  depression 102, 294–95
  friends 9
  grief 85–86
  myths 307–16
  prevention 317–24
  questions 304–5
  statistics **287**, **290**, 303
  warning signs 286–88, 294, 297–301,
    321–23

Suicide Awareness\Voices of Education
(SA\VE), contact information 292, 380
Suicide Information and Education Centre
(SIEC) 317n
contact information 292, 320, 380
Suicide Prevention Advocacy Network
(SPAN), contact information 292, 380
support groups 343–52
divorce 78
family issues 92
mental health care 331
panic disorder 190
personality disorders 233
supportive psychotherapy 175
surgery, anxiety disorders treatment 175–76
symptomatology, defined 354
systematic desensitization
defined 186
phobias 200
system of care, described 104

T

Tagamet (cimetidine) 171
TAG: Teen Age Grief, Inc.
contact information 88, 380
publications 83n
talk therapy, anxiety disorders treatment
175
taphephobia 195
tatoos 254
TCA see tricyclic antidepressants
"Teenagers commonly question the why
and how of suicide" (Barr) 303n
"Teenage Suicide" (NAMI) 285n
"Teen Eating Disorders" (NMHA) 241n
"Teen Self-Esteem: Feeling Good About
Yourself" (NMHA) 11n
"Teen Stress: A Teen's Guide to Surviving
Stress" (NMHA) 45n
Tegretol (carbamazepine) 140, 358
Tenormin (atenolol) 172, 197, **198**
teratophobia 195
tests
anger intensity 37
anxiety disorders **164**, 166
bipolar disorder 133
social phobia **208–9**

thalassophobia 195
thanatophobia 195
theophobia 195
therapeutic parenting, bipolar disorder
142–43
tiagabine 141
tics
defined 149
treatment 168
Tofranil (imipramine) 112, 170, 356
Topamax (topiramate) 141
topiramate 141
topophobia 195
Tourette's syndrome
bipolar disorder 134
defined 149
nerve abnormalities 156
toxicophobia 195
transcranial magnetic stimulation, bipolar
disorder 142
tranylcypromine 170, **198**, 200
trauma
anxiety disorders 157
post-traumatic stress disorder 216
trichotillomania
body dysmorphic disorder **250**
defined 257
obsessive-compulsive disorders 161
Trichotillomania Learning Center, contact
information 380
tricyclic antidepressants (TCA) 112, 170,
356, 361
triskaidekaphobia 195
12 Step Cyber Cafe, website 381
twins studies, suicidal behavior 312

U

University of Illinois
Champaign-Urbana Counseling Center
89n, **91**
US Department of Health and Human
Services (DHHS)
depression statistics 109
publications 3n

V

Vaknin, Sam 232
Valium (diazepam) 171, 197, **198**
valproic acid 140, 358
venlafaxine 108, 169
verapamil 141
verbal abuse 55–68, **62**
violence
  relationships 56–68
  stress 47
Vivactil 356

W

Wallace, Mike 115
weight lifting 19
weight loss, body image 21
Wellbutrin (bupropion) 108, 112, 357
"The Well-Connected Guide to Anxiety"
  (Nidus Information Services, Inc.)
  147n
"What Medications Are Used to Treat
  Anxiety Disorders" 353n
When Kids Hate Their Bodies (Pomice) 19
"When Your Parent Has A Mental Illness"
  (University of Illinois) 89n
"Why Am I So Sad?" (Nemours Founda-
  tion) 25n

Women for Sobriety, Inc., contact information 387
wrestling 19

X

Xanax (alprazolam) 141, 171, 197, **198**
xenophobia **195**

Y

Yellow Ribbon Suicide Prevention Program, contact information 292, 380
yoga
  anger control 39
  anxiety disorders treatment 168
  defined **36**
  depression 114
"You and Mental Health: What's the
  Deal?" (DHHS) 3n
"yo-yo dieting" 21

Z

zelophobia **195**
Zoloft (sertraline) 108, 112, 168, **198**, 200,
  201, 221, 251, 357
zoophobia **195**, 196
Zyprexa 141